Normal Findings in CT and MRI

Torsten B. Moeller, M.D.
Am Caritas-Krankenhaus
Dillingen/Saar
Germany

Emil Reif, M.D.
Am Caritas-Krankenhaus
Dillingen/Saar
Germany

210 Illustrations

T0261077

Thieme
Stuttgart · New York 2000

Library of Congress Cataloging-in-Publication Data

Moeller, Torsten B.
 [CT- und MRT-Normalbefunde. English]
 Normal findings in CT and MRI / Torsten B. Moller, Emil Reif. p. cm.
 Includes bibliographical references and index.
 ISBN 0-86577-864-7 (TNY). – ISBN 3-13-116521-9 (GTV)
 1. Tomography. 2. Magnetic resonance imaging. 3. Reference values (Medicine)
 4. Human anatomy. I. Reif, Emil. II. Title.
 [DNLM: 1. Magnetic Resonance Imaging. 2. Tomography, X-Ray
Computed. WN 185 M726c 1999a]
RC78.7.T6M6413   1999
616.07'57–dc21
DNLM/DLC   99-33663
for Library of Congress   CIP

© 2000 Georg Thieme Verlag,
Rüdigerstrasse 14,
D-70469 Stuttgart, Germany
Thieme New York, 333 Seventh Avenue,
New York, NY 10001, USA

Typesetting by primustype R. Hurler GmbH, D-73274 Notzingen, Germany typeset on Textline/HerculesPro
Cover design by Cyclus, Stuttgart
Printed in Germany by
Offizin Andersen Nexö, Leipzig

ISBN 3-13-116521-9 (GTV)
ISBN 0-86577-864-7 (TNY)
            1 2 3 4 5 6

Important Note: Medicine is an ever-changing science undergoing continual development. Research and clinical experience are continually expanding our knowledge, in particular our knowledge of proper treatment and drug therapy. Insofar as this book mentions any dosage or application, readers may rest assured that the authors, editors, and publishers have made every effort to ensure that such references are in accordance with **the state of knowledge at the time of production of the book.**

Nevertheless, this does not involve, imply, or express any guarantee or responsibility on the part of the publishers in respect to any dosage instructions and forms of application stated in the book. **Every user is requested to examine carefully** the manufacturer's leaflets accompanying each drug and to check, if necessary in consultation with a physician or specialist, whether the dosage schedules mentioned therein or the contraindications stated by the manufacturers differ from the statements made in the present book. Such examination is particularly important with drugs that are either rarely used or have been newly released on the market. Every dosage schedule or every form of application used is entirely at the user's own risk and responsibility. The authors and publishers request every user to report to the publishers any discrepancies or inaccuracies noticed.

To my father, Alfred Moeller,
in love and gratitude

Preface

This book, like its conventional counterpart *Normal Findings in Radiography*, deals with the apparently banal subject of the normal. It addresses the question of how to recognize what is normal and how to describe normal findings. These questions are as important in computed tomography and magnetic resonance imaging as in other modalities. Even "sectional imaging" is based on the classical approach of reading images and formulating findings.

This book follows the same format used in *Normal Findings in Radiography*. Each section starts with a brief descriptive interpretation of normal findings in the region of interest. Next comes a checklist that follows the sequence of the descriptive text and provides a systematic framework for image interpretation. Some of the checklist entries offer phrasing suggestions that may be helpful in the formulation of findings. Most sections conclude with a table of "Important Data" listing the normal ranges of values for the most important measurable parameters.

Of course, the "normal findings" presented here can only assist the radiologist in formulating his or her own findings. But regardless of whether we are taking a brief look or conducting a detailed evaluation, the system that is used in radiological interpretation should be reflected in the clarity and precision of the findings. This book is intended to further that goal.

We express sincere thanks to Alexandra Kläser, Sabine Mattil, Tanja Metzger, Monjuri Paul, Pia Saar-Schneider, Gisela Wagner, and especially Brigitte Schild for their help in compiling the CT and MR images. We also thank our colleagues Dr. Markus Bach, Dr. Christoph Buntru, Dr. Wolfgang Theobald, Dr. Albert Schmitt, Dr. Karl-Ernst Schmitt, Dr. Heike Rochelmayer, Dr. Pattrick Rosar, Dr. Lutger Henke, Dr. Klaus Kuhnen, and Dr. Christa Weller-Schweizer for their help and many suggestions, which helped see the book to its completion.

Dillingen, 1999

Torsten B. Moeller
Emil Reif

Table of Contents

Computed Tomography

CT: Head and Neck

Neurocranium

The interhemispheric fissure is centered on the midline. The cerebrum and cerebellum show normal cortical sulcation.

The cerebral ventricles are of normal size and symmetrically arranged. There are no signs of increased intracranial pressure.

Normal development of the white matter and cortex, with normal density of the periventricular white matter.

The basal ganglia, internal capsule, corpus callosum, and thalamus appear normal.

The brain stem and cerebellum, if evaluable, also appear normal.

Sella and pituitary are normal. Parasellar structures are unremarkable. There are no abnormalities in the cerebellopontine angle areas on both sides.

The paranasal sinuses and mastoid air cells are normally developed, clear, and pneumatized. The orbital contents are unremarkable. There are no abnormalities in the calvarium.

Interpretation

Normal cranial CT.

Checklist

Interhemispheric fissure
- Centered on the midline
- No displacement
- Falx cerebri:
  - Width
  - Density (no calcifications)

Cortical sulcation
- Of cerebrum and cerebellum (arbor vitae):
  - Configuration
  - Number of sulci
  - Width of sulci
  - No coarsening of sulci
  - No circumscribed narrowing or expansion
  - Well-defined cisterns and cortical markings

Cerebral cortex	• Width
	• Distribution (no ectopic tissue)
	• Density (see below), no calcifications or hemorrhages
	• No separation from the calvarium
	• No abnormal fluid collection (convex or concave) between the cerebral cortex and calvarium
Ventricles	• Shape
	• Size appropriate for age (see below)
	• Symmetry (no unilateral or circumscribed enlargement)
	• No signs of increased intracranial pressure (e.g., effaced sulci, narrowing or unilateral expansion of ventricles)
White matter	• Density (homogeneous, especially at periventricular sites—see below)
	• No hypodensities (circumscribed, lacunar, or diffuse)
	• No hyperdense changes (calcification, hemorrhage)
	• Normal width in relation to cortex
Basal ganglia, internal and external capsule, thalamus	• Position
	• Size
	• Delineation
	• Density
Corpus callosum	• Configuration
	• Size
	• Density
Brain stem	• Shape
	• Density (homogeneous)
	• No focal abnormalities
Cerebellum	• General form (symmetry)
	• Cortex (width, sulcation)
	• White matter (homogeneous density)
Intracranial vessels	• Course
	• Width
	• No abnormal dilatation
	• No vascular malformations
Sella and pituitary	• Size (see below)
	• Configuration
	• Density
	• Borders
	• Parasellar structures

Petrous pyramids
- Cerebellopontine angle area:
  - Width and symmetry of bony portions of internal auditory canals (see below)
  - CSF spaces symmetrical and of normal size, no masses
- Mastoid air cells, mastoid antrum
  - Anatomy
  - Pneumatization
  - Borders (wall thickness, smooth contours with no discontinuities)
  - No masses
  - No fluid-dense opacification
- Cochlea and semicircular canals:
  - Anatomy
  - Configuration
  - Smooth borders

Paranasal sinuses
- Anatomy
- Pneumatization
- Borders (wall thickness, smooth and continuous contours)
- Nasal cavity:
  - Pneumatization
  - Septum on midline
  - Turbinates (presence of superior, middle, and inferior turbinates; width)

Orbit
- Configuration of orbital cone
- Contents:
  - Globe (position—see below; size, density, wall thickness)
  - Eye muscles (position, course, density, width)
  - Optic nerve (course, width—see below)
  - Ophthalmic vein (course, width—see below)

Calvarium
- Configuration
- Contours (smooth, sharp, no expansion or bony outgrowths, no osteolytic or osteoplastic areas)

Important Data

Normal attenuation values: White matter   Cortex
- Noncontrast: 39 HU   32 HU
- Postcontrast: 41 HU   33 HU

(Each value has a deviation of ± 2 HU [Hounsfield units].)
Attenuation difference between cortex and white matter: approximately 7 HU

Ventricular dimensions

1 **Cella media index:**
   - B/A > 4 = normal
2 **Frontal horn of lateral ventricle (at level of foramen of Monro):**
   - Under age 40: < 12 mm
   - Over age 40: < 15 mm
3 **Width of third ventricle:**
   - < 5 mm in children (slightly more in infants)
   - < 7 mm in adults under age 60
   - < 9 mm in adults over age 60
4 **Width of ophthalmic vein:**
   - 3–4 mm
5 **Optic nerve (axial plane):**
   a Retrobulbar segment: 5.5 mm ± 0.8 mm
   b Narrowest point (at approximately midorbit): 4.2 mm ± 0.6 mm
6 **Position of globe:**
   - Posterior margin of globe is 9.9 mm ± 1.7 mm behind the interzygomatic line

Pituitary: Height of pituitary in sagittal reconstruction: 2–7 mm
Caution: normal size variations during:
             — Pregnancy: up to 12 mm
             — Puberty: up to 10 mm in girls, up to 8 mm in boys

Internal auditory canal: 5–10 mm (average 7.6 mm); should be ≤ 1 mm difference between the right and left sides

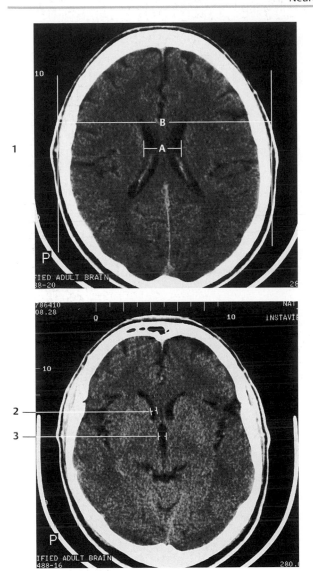

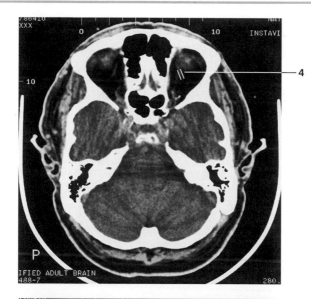

4

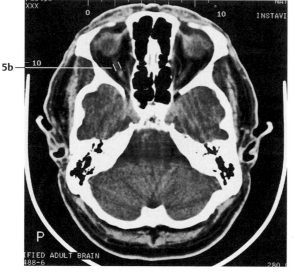

5b

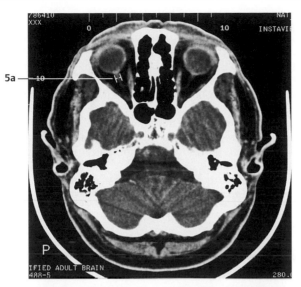

5a

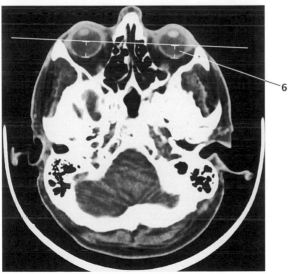

6

Pituitary

The sella shows normal size, position, and configuration. The borders of its floor and walls are smooth and sharply defined.

The pituitary shows normal position, shape, and size. The pituitary tissue shows normal, homogeneous density both before and after contrast administration. It contains no circumscribed hypodense or hyperdense areas.

The infundibulum is centered and of normal size.

The optic chiasm and suprasellar CSF spaces appear normal. The cavernous sinus and imaged portions of the internal carotid artery and carotid siphon are unremarkable.

Evaluable portions of the neurocranium show no abnormalities.

The sphenoid sinus is clear and pneumatized.

Interpretation

The pituitary appears normal.

Important Data

1 **Pituitary:**
   a Height (in the midcoronal plane): 2–7 mm
   Caution: allow for normal size variations during:
   • Pregnancy: up to 12 mm
   • Puberty: up to 10 mm in girls, up to 8 mm in boys
   b Width (transverse extent in coronal plane, women of childbearing age): 12.9 mm ± 1.6 mm
   Area of the pituitary in the coronal plane (height x width, women of childbearing age): 93 mm^2 ± 1.6 mm^2

2 **Optic chiasm:**
   • Coronal: a, width 9–18 mm; b, height 3–6 mm
   • Axial: c, width 12–27 mm; d, depth 4–9 mm

3 **Pituitary stalk:**
   • < 4 mm

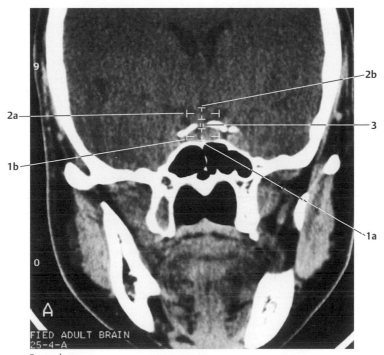

Coronal scan

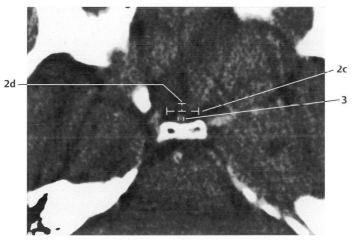

Axial scan

Checklist

Sella	• Position
	• Configuration (U shape)
	• Walls steep, not splayed, of normal size
	• Normal width of floor and walls
	• Borders smooth and sharp
Pituitary	• Position:
	— At the center of the sella
	• Configuration:
	— Bean-shaped
	— Superior border straight or slightly concave (convex only during puberty or pregnancy)
	• Size (see below)
	• Density:
	— Pituitary tissue homogeneous on noncontrast scans
	— Homogeneous contrast enhancement
	— No circumscribed hypodense or hyperdense areas within the pituitary
Infundibulum	• Position (centered)
	• Size (see below)
Optic chiasm	• Position
	• Size (see below)
	• Symmetry
	• Course of optic nerve
Suprasellar CSF spaces (chiasmatic cistern)	• Shape (symmetrical)
	• Width (no circumscribed narrowing)
Cavernous sinus	• Shape (symmetrical)
	• Size (see below)
	• No infiltration
Internal carotid artery (siphon area)	• Size
	• Course
	• Density
Neurocranium	• Temporal lobe
	• Hypothalamus
	• Floor of third ventricle
Sphenoid sinus	• Borders: smooth, normal width (especially of roof), contours
	• Pneumatization

Petrous Pyramids

The petrous pyramids are normally developed and symmetrical. They have smooth, intact cortical margins and a normal trabecular structure. The internal auditory canal is smooth and sharply defined on each side, with normal shape and diameter. The cochlea and semicircular canals appear normal. The mastoid air cells are normally developed, clear and pneumatized. Their bony walls are of normal thickness. The tympanic cavity is normally developed, and the auditory ossicles have a normal appearance.

Configuration of the cerebellopontine angle area on each side is normal, with clear delineation of the cerebellopontine angle cistern. The brain stem has normal configuration and CT density.

The external auditory canal appears normal on each side.

Other visualized portions of the neurocranium show no abnormalities.

Interpretation

Both petrous pyramids appear normal at CT.

Checklist

Petrous pyramids	• Configuration
	• Shape (triangular)
	• Bilateral symmetry
	• Delineation (cortical margins smooth and sharp)
	• Trabecular internal structure (no fracture lines, no bone destruction or circumscribed hypodense or hyperdense areas)
	• Smooth, sharp boundary with the calvarium (sinodural angle)
Internal auditory canals	• Shape
	• Course
	• Width (see below)
	• Bony boundaries (smooth, sharp)
	• Vestibulocochlear nerve (cranial nerve VIII) and facial nerve (cranial nerve VII), if visualized:
	— Width (uniform, no right-left disparity)
	— Enhancement characteristics (nonenhancing)
Cochlea and semicircular canals	• Anatomy
	• Configuration
	• Smooth borders

- Tympanic cavity:
  - Anatomy
  - Shape
  - Borders
  - Pneumatization
- Auditory ossicles (malleus, incus, stapes: presence, shape, relative positions in ossicular chain)

Mastoid
- Cellular anatomy (antrum, retrofacial cells, peritubal cells, peribulbar cells, marginal cells, terminal cells):
  - Cells small, large, or of mixed sizes; normal = uniform enlargement of cells from antrum to terminal cells)
  - Pneumatization
  - Borders (septal thickness, smooth contours with no discontinuities)
  - No masses
  - Not opacified by abnormal fluid or soft-tissue density

Cerebellopontine angle area
- Brain stem
  - Shape
  - Density (homogeneous)
  - No focal abnormalities
- Vestibulocochlear and facial nerve nuclei:
  - No hypodensity
  - No masses
- Entry sites of vestibulocochlear nerve (enters pons and medulla at lateral extension of medullopontine sulcus) and facial nerve:
  - Bilaterally symmetrical
- CSF spaces:
  - Cerebellopontine angle cistern (symmetrical, fluid density)
  - No masses
  - Well delineated
  - No vascular loop
- External auditory canals:
  - Anatomy
  - Course
  - Width
  - Borders

Rest of neurocranium	• Cerebrum (especially the temporal lobe) and cerebellum: — Configuration — Sulcation — Cortical markings (arbor vitae) well defined — Width of sulci — No circumscribed widening or narrowing — Homogeneous density of cortex and white matter (no hypodense or hyperdense changes)
CSF spaces	• Prepontine cistern • Fourth ventricle

Important Data

1 Internal auditory canal:
  • Approx. 5–10 mm, with ca. 1 mm difference between the right and left sides

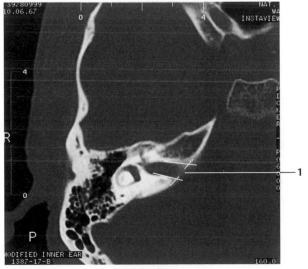

Axial scan through the internal auditory canal

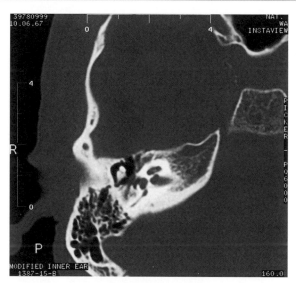

Axial scan for evaluating the auditory ossicles

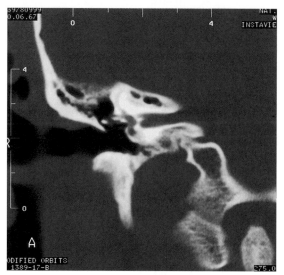

Coronal scan through the internal auditory canal

Orbit

The orbits are symmetrical and of normal size, with normal development of the orbital cone. The configuration of the smooth, sharply defined orbital walls is normal. There are no foci of bone destruction and there is no circumscribed widening of bony or soft-tissue components of the orbital walls.

The globes are symmetrical and show normal size and position. The ocular contents are of normal density. The ocular wall is smooth, sharply defined, and of normal thickness. The optic nerve shows a normal course and caliber on each side.

The eye muscles are normally positioned and display normal width and course. The retrobulbar fat and ophthalmic vein are unremarkable.

Imaged portions of the neurocranium and paranasal sinuses show no abnormalities.

Interpretation

The orbit and its contents appear normal.

Checklist

Orbits	• Symmetrical
	• Normal size
	• Normal orbital cone
Orbital walls	• Smooth, sharp borders
	• No bone destruction
	• No circumscribed widening of bone or soft-tissue components
Globe	• Position (see below)
	• Symmetry
	• Size (see below)
	• Spherical
Ocular contents	• Density
Ocular wall	• Borders (smooth and sharp)
	• Uniform thickness
Optic nerve	• Normal caliber (see below)
	• Course
Eye muscles	• Position
	• Width (see below)
	• Course
Retrobulbar fat	• Clear
	• No masses

Ophthalmic vein	• Course
	• Caliber (see below)
Lacrimal gland	• Size
	• Symmetry
	• No unilateral or bilateral enlargement
	• Position (see below)
	• No excavation or destruction of adjacent bone
	• Homogeneous internal structure
	• No hypodense areas
	• Smooth borders
Neurocranium	• Temporal lobes
	• Frontal lobes
Paranasal sinuses	• Maxillary sinuses
	• Ethmoid cells

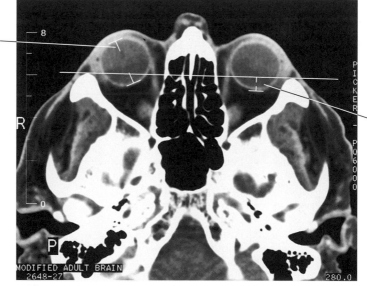

Axial scan

Important Data

1 Diameter of globe:
- Axial plane:
  - Right: 28.6 ± 1.2 mm
  - Left: 29.4 ± 1.4 mm
- Sagittal plane (reconstruction):
  - Right: 27.8 ± 1.2 mm
  - Left: 28.2 ± 1.2 mm

2 Position of globe:
- Posterior margin is 9.9 mm ± 1.7 mm behind the interzygomatic line

3 Optic nerve (axial plane):
- **a** Retrobulbar segment: 5.5 mm ± 0.8 mm
- **b** Narrowest point (at approximately mid-orbit): 4.2 mm ± 0.6 mm

4 Ophthalmic vein:
- 1.8 mm ± 0.5 mm (axial plane, 4 mm slice thickness)
- 2.7 mm ± 1 mm (coronal plane)

5 Eye muscles
- **a** Superior rectus: 3.8 mm ± 0.7 mm
- **b** Oblique: 2.4 mm ± 0.4 mm
- **c** Lateral rectus: 2.9 mm ± 0.6 mm
- **d** Medial rectus: 4.1 mm ± 0.5 mm
- **e** Inferior rectus: 4.9 mm ± 0.8 mm

Lacrimal gland: less than half of the gland is anterior to the frontozygomatic process.

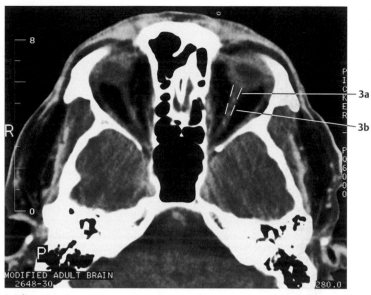

Axial scan

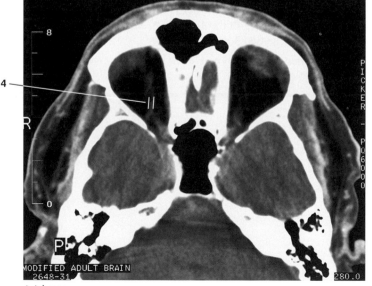

Axial scan

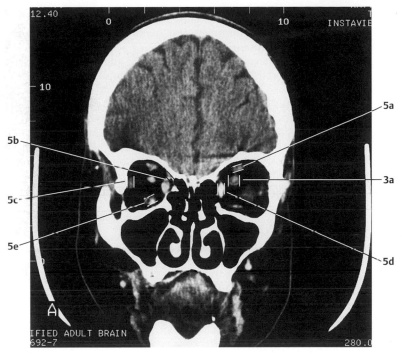

Coronal scan

Paranasal Sinuses

The frontal sinuses are normally developed, clear and pneumatized with smooth wall contours.

The ethmoid cells have a normal appearance and intact bony walls, especially on the orbital side. There are no areas of wall erosion or mucosal thickening.

The sphenoid sinus is normally developed and has a coarse honeycomb structure. There are no fluid collections or mucosal swelling.

The maxillary sinuses are bilaterally symmetrical and have smooth walls of normal thickness. The sinuses are clear and aerated with no bone destruction. The nasal septum is on the midline, and the turbinates are normally developed.

The nasal cavity, pharynx, and imaged parapharyngeal structures show no abnormalities.

Interpretation

The paranasal sinuses appear normal.

Checklist

Frontal sinuses	• Anatomy
	• Wall contours (smooth)
	• Pneumatization
Ethmoid cells	• Anatomy
	• Pneumatization
	• Bony structures (especially bordering the orbit: boundaries are smooth, sharp, and intact)
	• No wall erosions
	• No mucosal thickening
Sphenoid sinus	• Anatomy (coarse honeycomb structure)
	• Clear and pneumatized
	• No fluid collection
	• No mucosal swelling
	• Bony structures (smooth, intact walls, no erosion)
	• No extrinsic wall indentations
Maxillary sinuses	• Anatomy
	• Size (bilaterally symmetrical)
	• Bony structures (smooth, intact contours, walls of normal width, no bone erosion or destruction)
	• Pneumatization
	• No tooth roots projecting through maxillary sinus floor
Nasal cavity	• Anatomy (symmetry)
	• Size
	• Aeration (clear)
	• Nasal septum on the midline
	• Nasal turbinates (three on each side: superior, middle, inferior) are normally developed
Pharynx and parapharyngeal structures	• Anatomy (symmetry)
	• Size
	• Wall thickness
	• No foreign bodies, calcifications, or masses

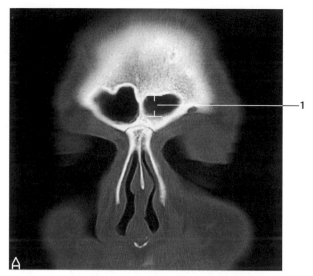

Coronal scan

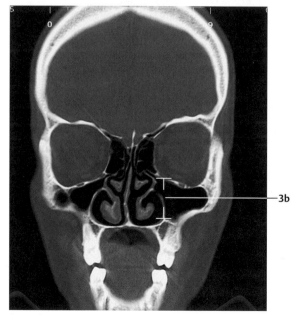

Coronal scan

Important Data

1 Frontal sinus:
- Height ca. 1.5–2 cm

2 Sphenoid sinus:
- Width 0.9–1.4 cm

3 Maxillary sinuses:
- **a** Width ca. 2 cm
- **b** Height ca. 2 cm

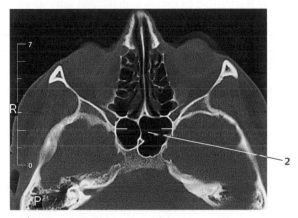

Axial scan

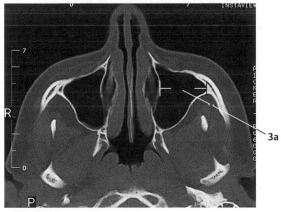

Axial scan

Cervical Soft Tissues

The cervical soft tissues show normal configuration, and the cervical spine is normally positioned.

The oral floor muscles are bilaterally symmetrical and normally developed. The spaces of the oral floor and neck are clear and well defined.

Imaged portions of the parotid and submandibular glands show no abnormalities.

The pharynx and larynx show normal boundaries and normal wall thickness.

The thyroid gland shows reasonable symmetry and normal size. The thyroid lobes have a normal internal structure.

Cervical vessels that can be evaluated with CT have a normal appearance.

The muscular structures of the neck appear normal, and there are no signs of cervical lymphadenopathy.

Interpretation

The cervical soft tissues appear normal.

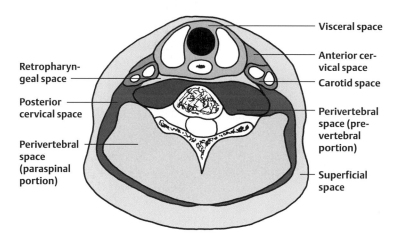

Retropharyngeal space

Posterior cervical space

Perivertebral space (paraspinal portion)

Visceral space

Anterior cervical space

Carotid space

Perivertebral space (prevertebral portion)

Superficial space

Checklist

Cervical soft tissues	• Configuration
	• Normal anatomy
	• Normal position of cervical spine
Oral floor muscles	• Anatomy
	• Width
	• Bilateral symmetry
	• Boundary definition
	• Internal structure
	• Spaces of oral floor are clearly defined
Submandibular gland (and parotid gland)	• Size (symmetry)
	• Density
	• No dilatation of glandular duct
	• No hypodense or hyperdense areas within the glandular tissue
Pharynx and larynx	• Shape (symmetrical)
	• Size
	• Smooth walls
	• Normal wall thickness
	• No masses
Cervical spaces	• Retropharyngeal space
	• Parapharyngeal space (visceral space)
	• Carotid space
	• Anterior and posterior cervical spaces
	• Perivertebral space (prevertebral and paraspinal portions):
	— Configuration
	— Boundaries
	— Symmetry
	— Internal structure
	— Width (see below)
Esophagus	• Position
	• Wall thickness (see below)
	• Boundaries
	• No masses
Thyroid gland	• Anatomy (two lobes, largely symmetrical)
	• Size (see below)
	• Internal structure (homogeneous)
	• No cysts
	• No nodules
	• No calcifications

Cervical vessels	• Course
	• Caliber (see below)
	• No abrupt caliber changes
	• No calcifications
Neck muscles	• Anatomy
	• Symmetry
	• Borders
	• Internal structure
Lymph node stations	• No lymphadenopathy
Cervical spine (if evaluable)	• Vertebral bodies
	— Number
	— Shape
	— Position
	— Contours
	• Intervertebral disk spaces
	• Spinal canal:
	— Width
	— No circumscribed narrowing
	• Normal width of cervical spinal cord
	• No masses
	• No narrowing

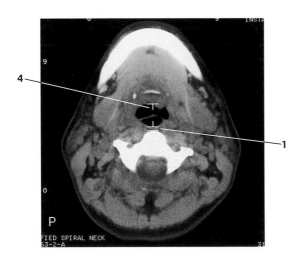

Important Data

Prevertebral soft tissues
1 Retropharyngeal: ca. 1.7 ± 0.7 mm
2 Retroglottic: ca. 6.0 ± 1.1 mm
3 Retrotracheal: ca. 8.4 ± 2.5 mm

Lumina of upper respiratory tract (normal respiration):
4 Laryngeal inlet (hyoid level): ca. 19 ± 4 mm
5 Glottis: ca. 21 ± 4 mm
6 Trachea: ca. 17 ± 3 mm
7 Thyroid dimensions:
  a Length: 3.6–6 cm (reconstruction)
  b Width: 1.5–2 cm
  c Depth: 1–2 cm

Vascular calibers (at level of thyroid gland)
8 Common carotid artery: 6–10 mm
9 **Esophagus:** wall thickness 3 mm

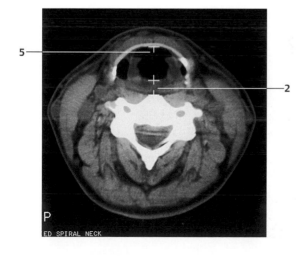

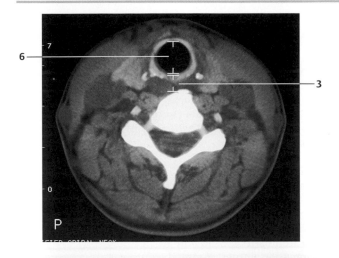

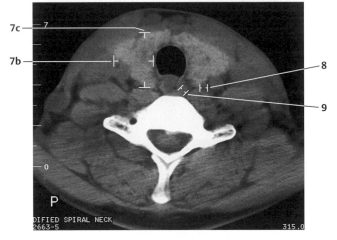

CT: Chest

Thoracic Organs

Both lungs are normally aerated and are applied to the chest wall on all sides. There is no sign of circumscribed pleural thickening and no fluid collection.

Pulmonary structure is normal and shows normal vascular markings. There are no intrapulmonary nodules or patchy opacities.

The mediastinum is centered and of normal width. There is no evidence of masses in the anterior, central, or posterior compartments.

The hilar region on each side is unremarkable, and the main bronchi appear normal.

The heart is orthotopic with normal configuration. The cardiac chambers are of normal size.

Major intrathoracic vessels and imaged portions of the supra-aortic vessels are unremarkable.

The thoracic skeleton and thoracic soft tissues show no abnormalities.

Interpretation

The thoracic organs appear normal at CT.

Checklist

Lungs
- Anatomy (paired and symmetrical)
- Fully apposed to the chest wall
- No pleural thickening
- No wall thickening
- No fluid collection (patchy or circumscribed)
- Complete aeration
- Normal attenuation values of lung parenchyma (see below)
- Pulmonary structure
- Vascular markings (diminish from center to periphery)
- No pulmonary nodules
- No patchy opacities (e.g., plaques or infiltrates)

Mediastinum	• Configuration, position:
	− Centered
	− Width (see below)
	− No masses in the anterior, central, or posterior compartment
	• Hilar region:
	− No masses or lymphadenopathy
	• Main bronchi:
	− Anatomy
	− Course
	− Width (see below)
	• Heart:
	− Position (centered slightly left of midline)
	− Configuration
	− Size (cardiac chambers−see below)
	− Myocardium (width−see below)
Vessels	• Intrathoracic vessels (ascending aorta, aortic arch, descending aorta, vena cava−see below):
	− Anatomy
	− Size
	• Supra-aortic vessels (subclavian artery, brachiocephalic trunk, left common carotid artery):
	− Anatomy
	− Size
Diaphragm	• Shape (no contour abnormalities, costophrenic angle is sharp and clear)
	• Position (approximately the level of the 10th–11th posterior rib)
	• Width (no circumscribed widening, no defect)
Thoracic skeleton (ribs, clavicle, sternum, scapula)	• Position
	• Structure
	• Contours and symmetry
	• No bony expansion or destruction
	• Thoracic spine:
	− Position
	− Shape of thoracic vertebrae
Thoracic soft tissues	• Configuration
	• Width
	• Symmetry
	• Density

Important Data

1 CT density of lung parenchyma:
- -403 ± 25 HU

2 Diameter of aorta:
- < 4 cm

a Ascending aorta:
- At level of pulmonary trunk bifurcation: 3.2 cm ± 0.5 cm
- At level of aortic root: 3.7 cm ± 0.3 cm

b Descending aorta:
- 2.5 cm ± 0.4 cm
- Aortic arch: 1.5 cm ± 1.2 cm

Ratio of ascending to descending aortic diameters = 1.5:1

3 Diameter of superior vena cava:
- At level of aortic arch: 1.4 cm ± 0.4 cm
- At level of pulmonary trunk bifurcation: 2 cm ± 0.4 cm

4 Diameter of pulmonary arteries:
- Pulmonary trunk: 2.4 cm ± 0.2 cm
- Proximal right pulmonary artery: 1.9 cm ± 0.3 cm
- Distal right pulmonary artery: 1.5 cm ± 0.3 cm
- Left pulmonary artery: 2.1 cm ± 0.4 cm

5 Width of main bronchi:
- Right ca. 15 mm
- Left ca. 13 cm

6 Mediastinum:
- Transverse diameter of thymus: 1–2 cm

Heart
Dimensions of cardiac chambers
7 Right atrium:
- Maximum transverse diameter: 4.4 cm
  - At level of aortic root: 1.9 cm ± 0.8 cm
  - At level of mitral valve: 3.2 cm ± 1.2 cm
  - At center of ventricles: 2.8 cm ± 0.4 cm

8 Left atrium:
a Maximum anteroposterior diameter: 4–5 cm
- At level of aortic root: 2.4 cm ± 4.5 cm
- At level of mitral valve: 2.9 cm ± 4.9 cm

b Maximum transverse diameter: 9 cm
- At level of aortic root: 5.5 cm ± 8.4 cm
- At level of mitral valve: 4.9 cm ± 9.1 cm

9 Angle between midsagittal plane and septum = 38°

10 **Thickness of ventricular septum:**
  • Approximately 5–10 mm
11 **Thickness of pericardium:**
  • 1–2 mm
12 **Thickness of myocardium:**
  • 10–12 mm

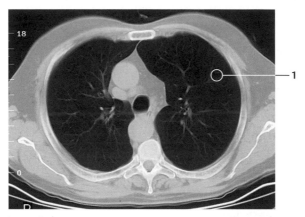

Lung window

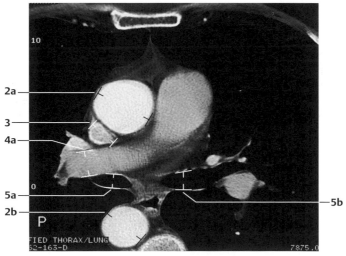

Contrast bolus scan at level of pulmonary trunk bifurcation

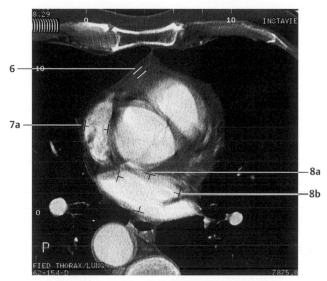

Contrast bolus scan at level of aortic root

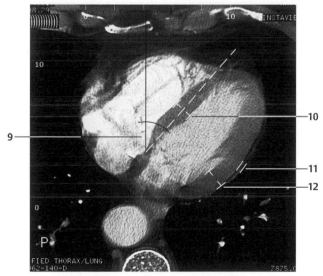

Contrast bolus scan through center of ventricles

CT: Abdomen

Upper Abdominal Organs

The liver is normally positioned and has normal size and smooth borders.

Its internal structure and attenuation values are normal. The intrahepatic and extrahepatic bile ducts and gallbladder are unremarkable.

The spleen is orthotopic and of normal size. It has smooth outer contours and a homogeneous internal structure.

The pancreas is normal in size, position, and internal structure with smooth, lobulated outer contours. The pancreatic duct is unobstructed.

Both kidneys show normal size and position. The renal parenchyma shows normal width and structure.

The renal pelvis and calices show a normal configuration. The urinary drainage tract is unobstructed.

The adrenal glands are unremarkable.

Major blood vessels appear normal, and there is no evidence of lymphadenopathy.

Imaged portions of the lung and soft tissues are normal.

Interpretation

The upper abdominal organs appear normal at CT.

Checklist

Liver

- Position
  - Directly below the right hemidiaphragm
- Size (see below)
- Borders:
  - Smooth
  - Sharp
- Normal attenuation values (see below)
- Homogeneous internal parenchymal structure
- No focal abnormalities
- Intrahepatic bile ducts:
  - Course (centrifugal)
  - Width (general rule: ducts should no longer

be visible after contrast administration—see below)
— No calculi
— No air

- Extrahepatic bile ducts:
  — Course (from porta hepatis to head of pancreas)
  — Width (see below)
  — Contents of homogeneous fluid density
  — No calculi
  — No air
- Gallbladder:
  — Size (see below)
  — Smooth outer contours
  — Normal wall thickness (see below)
  — No pericholecystic fluid
- Gallbladder contents:
  — Homogeneous
  — Fluid density
  — No calculi (hypodense or hyperdense)
  — No air
- Porta hepatis occupied by the hepatic artery, common bile duct, and portal vein
- No masses
- No lymphadenopathy
- Costophrenic sinus clear and aerated on both sides

Spleen
- Size (see below)
- Smooth outer contours
- Homogeneous internal structure
- Attenuation values (see below)

Pancreas
- Size normal for age (see below)
- Normal lobulation
- Smooth outer contours
- Pancreatic duct unobstructed
- No peripancreatic fluid
- Normal para-aortic region

Kidneys
- Paired
- Position (see below)
- Size (see below)
- Smooth contours
- Width of parenchyma (see below)
- Density (see below)

	• Width of cortex and medulla
	• Renal pelvis (anatomy, symmetry, size, no widening, contents of homogeneous fluid density)
	• Calices (shape, width, homogeneous contents)
	• Enhancement characteristics (see below)
Ureters	• Not duplicated
	• Course
	• No obstruction of urinary drainage
	• Normal-appearing periureteral fat
	• Near-simultaneous opacification of both ureters after contrast administration
Adrenal glands	• Shape
	• Size (see below)
	• Slender crura
	• No circumscribed hypodense (cyst, adenoma), isodense or hyperdense expansion
Intestinal structures (colon haustrations, small bowel)	• Anatomy
	• Shape
	• Wall thickness
	• Homogeneous opacification after oral contrast administration
	• No free extraintestinal or intra-abdominal air or fluid
Major vessels	• Position
	• Size (see below)
	• Luminal opacification after contrast administration
	• No large (intimal) calcifications
	• No mural thrombosis
	• No dissection
Lymph node stations (especially retrocrural, mesenteric, paraaortic)	• No lymphadenopathy
Lung segments	• Configuration
	• Complete aeration
	• No adhesions
	• No pulmonary nodules
Soft tissues	• Anatomy
	• Symmetry
	• Density

Important Data

Dimensions:

1 Liver:
  a Angle of left hepatic border: ca. 45°
  b Left lobe (anteroposterior diameter measured on the para-vertebral line): up to 5 cm
• Caudate lobe/right lobe (CL/RL) = 0.37 ± 0.16 (e.g., 0.88 ± 0.2 in cirrhosis)

2 Spleen:
  a Depth (D): 4–6 cm
  b Width (W): 7–10 cm
  c Length (L): 11–15 cm (reconstruction)
     Splenic index: D×W×L = between 160 and 440

3 Pancreas:
  a Head up to 3.5 cm
  b Body up to 2.5 cm
  c Tail up to 2.5 cm

4 Adrenal glands (variable):
• Crural thickness < 10 mm

5 Gallbladder:
  a Horizontal diameter up to 5 cm (> 5 cm is suspicious for hydrops)
  b Width of gallbladder wall:
     • 1–3 mm
  c Width of common bile duct:
     • ≤ 8 mm (after cholecystectomy: ≤ 10 mm)

6 Inferior vena cava:
• Transverse diameter up to 2.5 cm

7 Abdominal aorta:
• Transverse diameter ca. 18–30 mm

8 Kidneys:
  a Anteroposterior diameter ca. 4 cm
  b Transverse diameter 5–6 cm; craniocaudal diameter (= highest to lowest section) 8–13 cm
  c Transverse renal axis: posteriorly divergent angle of 120°
  d Width of renal cortex: 4–5 mm
  e Width of ureter: 4–7 mm

Position of superior poles of kidneys:
• Right: superior border of L1
• Left: inferior border of T12

Time to corticomedullary equilibrium:
- 1 minute

Contrast excretion into the pyelocaliceal system:
- 3 minutes

Gerota fascia (thickness):
- 1–2 mm

Lymph nodes larger than 1 cm are suspicious for pathology.

Attenuation values:
- Liver: 65 ± 10 HU
- Spleen: 45 ± 5 HU
- Pancreas: 40 ± 10 HU
- Fat: -65 to -100 HU
- Kidneys: 30–45 HU without contrast medium; renal cortex after contrast medium: approx. 140 HU
- Adrenal glands: 25–40 HU without contrast medium
- Muscle: 45 ± 5 HU
- Blood vessels: approx. 40–55 HU without contrast medium
- Gallbladder contents: 0–25 HU

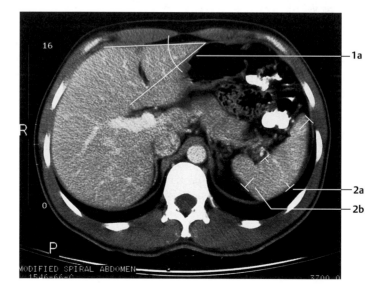

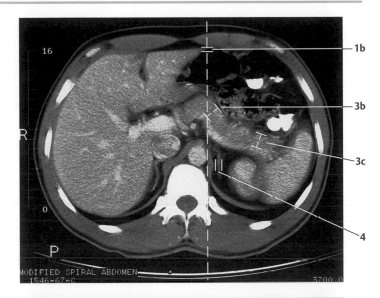

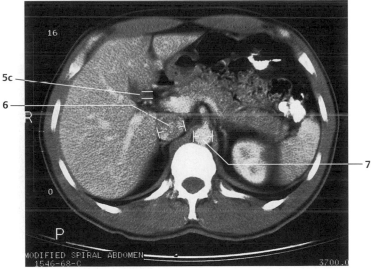

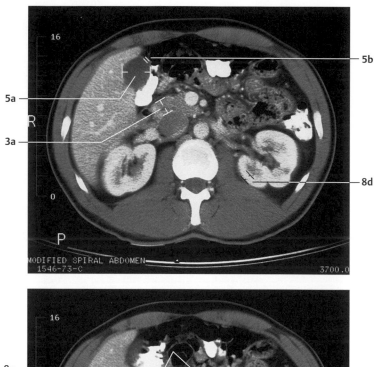

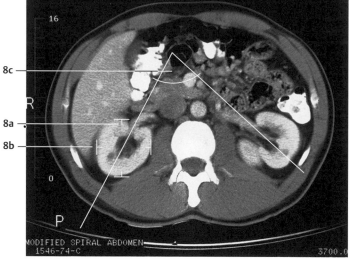

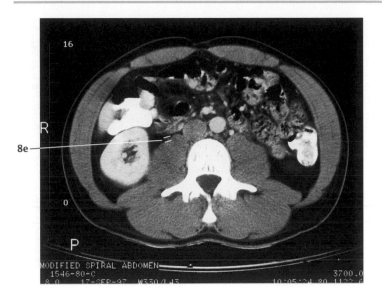

Liver

The liver is orthotopic and of normal size, with smooth borders and normal attenuation values. It presents a normal internal structure with no focal abnormalities.

The intrahepatic and extrahepatic bile ducts are normal in their course, width, and contents.

The gallbladder appears normal, presenting smooth borders and homogeneous contents.

The porta hepatis shows no abnormalities.

Other visualized upper abdominal organs are unremarkable.

Interpretation

The liver appears normal at CT.

Checklist

Liver
- Position:
  - Directly below the right hemidiaphragm
- Size (see below)
- Borders:
  - Smooth
  - Sharp
- Attenuation values (see below)
- Homogeneous internal parenchymal structure, no focal abnormalities
- Intrahepatic bile ducts:
  - Course (centrifugal)
  - Width (general rule: ducts should no longer be visible after contrast administration)
  - No calculi
  - No air
- Extrahepatic bile ducts:
  - Course (from porta hepatis to head of pancreas)
  - Width (see below)
  - Contents of homogeneous fluid density
  - No calculi
  - No air
- Gallbladder:
  - Size (see below)
  - Contours (smooth and sharp)
  - Wall thickness (see below; no general or circumscribed thickening)
  - No pericholecystic fluid
- Gallbladder contents:
  - Homogeneous
  - Fluid density (see below)
  - No calculi (hypodense or hyperdense)
  - No air
  - Porta hepatis occupied by the hepatic artery, common bile duct, and portal vein; no masses or lymphadenopathy
  - Costophrenic sinus clear and aerated on both sides; no pleural effusion, no infiltrates, no masses

Spleen	• Position
	• Configuration
	• Size (see below)
	• Density (homogeneous internal structure)
	• Contours (smooth)
Pancreas	• Position
	• Configuration
	• Size
	• Density (homogeneous internal structure)
	• Contours (smooth, lobulated)
	• Pancreatic duct
	• Para-aortic region unremarkable
Adrenal glands, kidneys (if visualized)	• Position
	• Size (see below)
	• Internal structure
Abdominal cavity	• Intestinal structures (if visualized and evaluable: configuration, width, wall thickness)
	• No free extraintestinal or intra-abdominal air or fluid
Soft tissues	

Important Data

Dimensions

1 Liver:
  a Angle of left hepatic border: ca. 45°
  b Caudate lobe/right lobe (CL/RL) = 0.37 ± 0.16 (e.g., 0.88 ± 0.2 in cirrhosis. Reference lines [from medial side]: line I is tangent to the medial border of the caudate lobe; line II is parallel to I and tangent to the lateral aspect of the portal vein; line III is tangent to the lateral hepatic border and perpendicular to a line midway between the portal vein and inferior vena cava and perpendicular to I and II.
  c Left lobe (anteroposterior diameter measured on the paravertebral line): up to 5 cm

2 Portal vein:
  • Up to 1.5 cm

3 Hepatic veins:
  • Up to 0.5 cm

4 **Gallbladder:**
- Horizontal diameter up to 5 cm (> 5 cm is suspicious for hydrops)

5 **Width of gallbladder wall:**
- 1–3 mm

6 **Width of common bile duct:**
- ≤ 8 mm (after cholecystectomy: ≤ 10 mm)

Spleen:
- Depth (D): 4–6 cm
- Width (W): 7–10 cm
- Length (L): 11–15 cm
- Splenic index: D×W×L = 160–440

Kidneys:
- Craniocaudal diameter: 8–13 cm
- Anteroposterior diameter: ca. 4 cm
- Transverse diameter 5–6 cm

Position of superior poles:
- Right: superior border of L1
- Left: inferior border of T12

Width of renal cortex:
- 4–5 mm

Gerota fascia (thickness):
- 1–2 mm

Adrenal glands (variable):
- Crural thickness < 10 mm

Diameter of abdominal aorta:
- Approximately 18–30 mm

Lymph nodes larger than 1 cm are suspicious for pathology.

Attenuation values
- Liver: 65 ± 10 HU
- Gallbladder contents: 0–25 HU
- Spleen: 45 ± 5 HU
- Pancreas: 40 ± 10 HU
- Fat: -65 to -100 HU
- Kidneys: 35–45 HU without contrast medium
- Adrenal glands: 25–40 HU without contrast medium
- Muscle: 45 ± 5 HU
- Blood vessels: ca. 40–55 HU without contrast medium

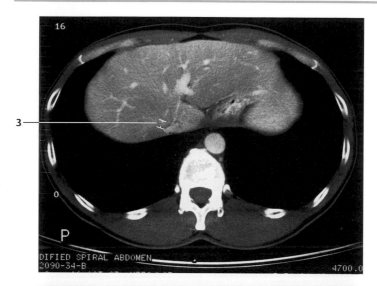

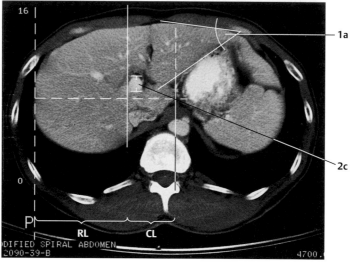

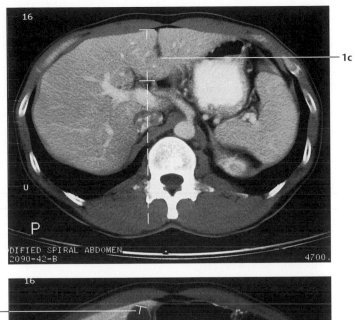

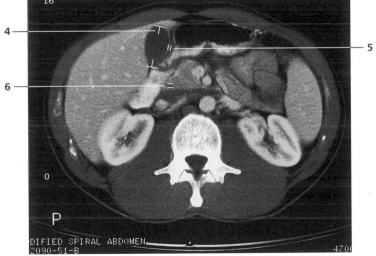

Pancreas

The pancreas is orthotopic and presents a normal size and smooth borders.

Lobulation of the pancreas is normal and appropriate for age. The parenchyma shows normal internal structure and attenuation values with no hypodense or hyperdense intrapancreatic changes. The pancreatic duct shows normal course and caliber.

The duodenal colon is unremarkable. The common bile duct is of normal width and has an unobstructed, fluid-filled lumen.

The visualized intrahepatic and extrahepatic bile ducts appear normal. No abnormalities appear in the peripancreatic fat.

The splenic vein and mesenteric vessels appear normal. The mesenteric root is normal.

Imaged portions of the liver, spleen, kidneys, and adrenals are unremarkable, as are the pararenal and paracolic spaces.

The major vessels appear normal, and there are no signs of lymphadenopathy.

Interpretation

The pancreas appears normal at CT.

Checklist

Pancreas
- Position
- Configuration
- Size appropriate for age (see below)
- Normal lobulation (borders are usually straight in adolescents and show increased lobulation with aging)
- Smooth outer contours
- Internal parenchymal structure (homogeneous in young patients, becomes slightly nonhomogeneous with aging)
- No focal abnormalities (e.g., calcifications, cysts, tumors)
- Pancreatic duct:
  - Position (centered in the pancreas)
  - Width (see below)
  - No obstruction
  - No circumscribed or beaded dilatation or narrowing

- — Termination (usually opens into duodenum at Vater papilla with intrapancreatic part of common bile duct)
- No peripancreatic fluid (exudate tracks along the left and right pararenal spaces, into the omental bursa, and along the paracolic gutters)
- Para-aortic region
- *Splenic vein:*
  - — Course (lies against posterior surface of pancreas, runs from splenic hilum to portal vein)
  - — Width
- Lymph nodes (especially the parapancreatic and pancreaticosplenic stations):
  - — Size
  - — Number
- Peripancreatic fat:
  - — Fat attenuation
  - — No infiltration
  - — No fluid
- *Mesenteric artery and vein:*
  - — Course
  - — Size
- Duodenum (descending part: directly adjacent to head of pancreas; horizontal part: directly adjacent to uncinate process)
- Transverse mesocolon
- *Stomach:*
  - — Smooth posterior surface
  - — Normal wall thickness
  - — Surrounded by fatty tissue
- Extrahepatic bile ducts:
  - — Course (from porta hepatis to head of pancreas)
  - — Width (see below)
  - — Contents of homogeneous fluid density
  - — No calculi
  - — No air

Liver
- Position
- Size (if evaluable)
- Borders
  - — Smooth
  - — Sharp

- Attenuation values (see below)
- Homogeneous internal parenchymal structure
- Intrahepatic bile ducts
  - Course (centrifugal)
  - Width (general rule: should no longer be visible after contrast administration)
- Gallbladder (if visualized):
  - Size
  - Contents
  - Wall thickness
- Porta hepatis occupied by the hepatic artery, common bile duct, and portal vein; no masses or lymphadenopathy

Spleen
- Position
- Size
- Borders
- Density (see below)

Kidneys
- Paired
- Position
- Size
- Smooth contours
- Width of parenchyma
- Density (see below)

Adrenal glands
- Shape
- Size (see below)
- Symmetrical crura
- No circumscribed expansion

Intestinal structures (colon haustrations, small bowel)
- Normal wall thickness
- Homogeneous opacification by oral contrast medium
- No free extraintestinal or intra-abdominal air or fluid

Blood vessels (aorta, inferior vena cava)
- Size
- No luminal obstruction

Lymph node stations (para-aortic, retro-crural)
- No lymphadenopathy

Important Data

Dimensions of pancreas (normal ranges for age):

Age (years)	Head 1 (mm)	Body 2 (mm)	Tail 3 (mm)
• 20–30	25–32	17–21	16–20
• 31–40	23–29	16–20	15–18
• 41–50	22–29	16–19	14–17
• 51–60	21–27	14–18	14–17
• 61–70	20–26	14–18	13–16
• 71–80	17–25	12–17	11–15

Rule of thumb: head ≤ 3.5 cm, body and tail ≤ 2.5 cm

4 Pancreatic duct:
  • Width 1–3 mm

5 Width of common bile duct:
  • ≤ 8 mm (≤ 10 mm after cholecystectomy)

Attenuation values:
  • Pancreas: 40 ± 10 HU
  • Liver: 65 ± 10 HU
  • Spleen: 45 ± 5 HU
  • Kidneys: 35–45 HU without contrast medium; renal cortex after contrast medium: ca. 140 HU
  • Adrenal glands: 25–40 HU without contrast medium
  • Muscle: 45 ± 5 HU
  • Blood vessels: ca. 40–55 HU without contrast medium
  • Gallbladder contents: 0–25 HU
  • Fat: -65 to -100 HU

Dimensions:
  • Spleen: width 7–10 cm, height 4–6 cm, length 11–15 cm
  • Adrenal glands (variable): crural thickness ≤ 10 mm
  • Gallbladder: horizontal diameter up to 5 cm (> 5 cm is suspicious for hydrops)
  • Width of gallbladder wall: 1–3 mm
  • Gerota fascia (thickness): 1–2 mm
  • Diameter of abdominal aorta: approx. 18–30 mm
  • Lymph nodes larger than 1 cm are suspicious for pathology.

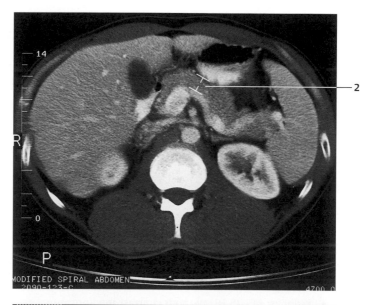

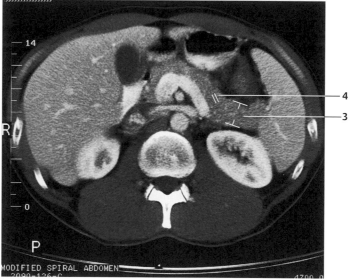

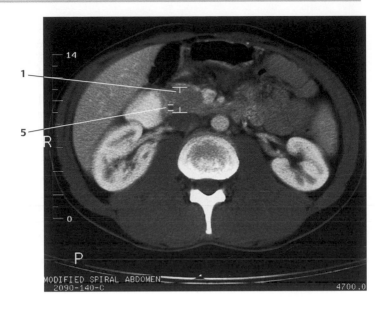

Kidneys

Both kidneys appear normal in size and position, with normal width and density of the renal parenchyma. There is no evidence of a mass. The calices are of normal shape. The renal pelvis is normal and free of stones, and there is no obstruction of urinary drainage.

Contrast-enhanced scans show a normal time to corticomedullary equilibrium and timely, symmetrical contrast excretion into the renal pelves with no filling defects.

The perirenal and pararenal spaces are unremarkable.

Other visualized upper abdominal organs, especially the adrenal glands, show no abnormalities.

Interpretation

Both kidneys appear normal at CT.

Checklist

Kidneys
- Anatomy:
  - Paired
  - Position (see below)
  - Size (see below)
- Organ contours:
  - Smooth and sharp
- Width of parenchyma
- Density (see below)
- Normal relation of cortex to medulla
- Renal pelves:
  - Structure and shape of caliceal groups
  - Bilateral symmetry
  - No expansion
- Ureters:
  - One per side
  - Course
  - Width (see below)
  - No obstruction
- Peri- and pararenal spaces:
  - Fat attenuation
  - No masses
  - No increase in soft-tissue structures
  - No fluid

	• Peri- and pararenal fasciae:
	– Course
	– Width (no diffuse or circumscribed thickening)
Adrenal glands	• Shape
	• Size (see below)
	• Slender crura
	• No circumscribed expansion
Retroperitoneal space	• No mass, fluid, or increased density
Intestinal structures	• Colon haustrations, small bowel
	• Wall thickness
	• Homogeneous contrast enhancement
	• No free extraintestinal or intra-abdominal air or fluid
Vessels	• Course
	• Size (see below)
	• No lymphadenopathy (see below)
Soft tissues	• Density
	• Symmetry
	• Muscles (size, internal structure, borders)
	• Fat (density, no soft-tissue or fluid infiltration)

Important Data

1 **Distance between renal poles:**
   - Superior poles: ca. 10 cm (4–16 cm) apart
   - Inferior poles: ca. 13 cm (9–18.5 cm) apart
2 **Transverse renal axis:**
   - Posteriorly divergent angle of 120°
3 **Transverse renal diameter at level of hilum:**
   - 5–6 cm (**a**, transverse) x 3–4 cm (**b**, anteroposterior)
4 **Width of cortex:**
   - 4–5 mm
5 **Width of ureter:**
   - 4–7 mm
6 **Gerota fascia (thickness):**
   - 1–2 mm
   Position of superior poles of kidneys:
   - Right: superior border of L1
   - Left: inferior border of T12 (variable; note that the difference does not exceed 1.5 vertebral body heights)
   Renal dimensions:
   - Craniocaudal (= highest to lowest section!) 8–13 cm
   Right–left disparity in renal sizes:
   - Craniocaudal < 1.5 cm
   Renal attenuation values:
   - 35–45 HU without contrast medium
   - Renal cortex ca. 140 HU after contrast administration
   Time to corticomedullary equilibrium:
   - 1 minute
   Contrast excretion into the pyelocaliceal system:
   - 3 minutes
7 **Size of adrenal glands (variable):**
   - Crural thickness < 10 mm
   Density of normal adrenal glands: 25–40 HU without contrast medium
8 **Abdominal aorta:**
   - Transverse diameter ca. 18–30 mm
9 **Inferior vena cava:**
   - Transverse diameter up to 2.5 cm
   Vascular density: ca. 40–55 HU without contrast medium
   Lymph nodes larger than 1 cm are suspicious for pathology.

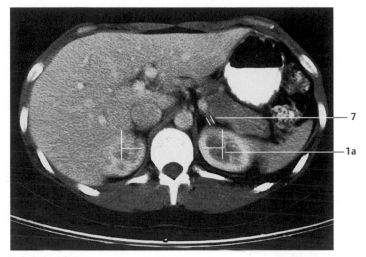

Early bolus phase

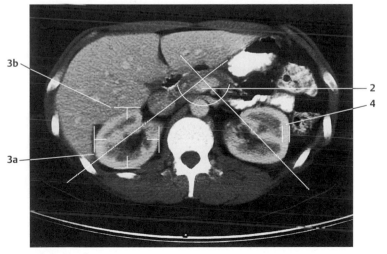

Early bolus phase

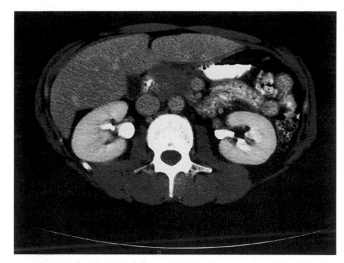

Late phase with corticomedullary equilibrium and opacification of the renal pelvis

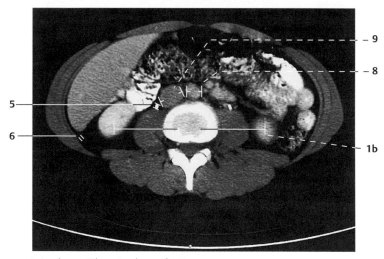

Late phase with ureteral opacification

Adrenal Glands

Both adrenal glands present normal size and position with normally developed crura. There is no evidence of a mass and no circumscribed expansion.

The adrenal compartment is unremarkable.

Postcontrast scans show normal adrenal enhancement characteristics and dynamics.

Other visualized upper abdominal organs, especially the kidneys, show no abnormalities.

Interpretation

Both adrenal glands appear normal at CT.

Checklist

Adrenal glands	• Paired
	• Position (superior and anterior to the kidneys)
	• Shape
	• Size (see below)
	• Borders (smooth, sharp)
	• Slender adrenal crura showing no circumscribed hypodense, isodense, or hyperdense expansion
	• No calcifications
	• Adrenal compartment:
	— Fat attenuation
	— No mass
	• Enhancement characteristics:
	— Uniform increase in density
	— No hypodense or hyperdense lesions within the adrenal crura
Liver	• Size (see below)
	• Borders:
	— Smooth
	— Sharp
	• Homogeneous internal parenchymal structure
	• Intrahepatic and extrahepatic bile ducts
	• Costophrenic sinus clear and aerated on each side
Spleen	• Size (see below)
	• Smooth outer contours
	• Homogeneous internal structure
Pancreas	• Size
	• Pancreatic duct

Kidneys	• Paired
	• Position (see below)
	• Size (see below)
	• Smooth contours
Stomach and bowel	• Position
	• Size
	• No masses
	• No infiltration
Major vessels	• Transverse diameter
	• Flow
Lymph nodes	• No lymphadenopathy
Diaphragm	• No circumscribed widening
	• Lungs in the costophrenic sinus (no effusion or opacities)
Vertebral bodies Soft tissues	• Margins, bony structure

Important Data

Dimensions

1 Adrenal glands (variable):
- Crural thickness < 10 mm
- Density (without contrast medium): 25–40 HU

Position of superior poles of kidneys:
- Right: superior border of L1
- Left: inferior border of T12

Transverse renal axis:
- Posteriorly divergent angle of 120°

Renal dimensions:
- Craniocaudal: 8–13 cm
- Anteroposterior: ca. 4 cm
- Transverse: 5–6 cm

Gerota fascia (thickness):
- 1–2 mm

Spleen:
- Width: 7–10 cm
- Depth: 4–6 cm
- Length: 11–15 cm

Diameter of abdominal aorta:
- Approximately 18–30 mm

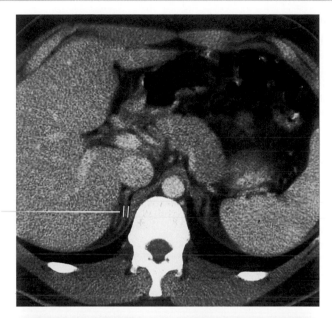

1 ——

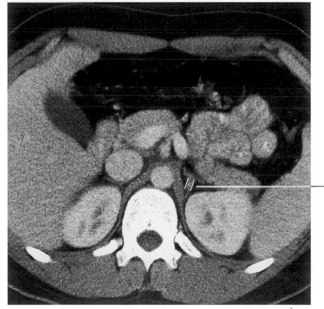

—— 1

Female Pelvis

The pelvic inlet appears normal, with normal configuration of the iliac wings and iliopsoas muscles.

Imaged bowel structures, especially the cecum and rectum, show no abnormalities with no evidence of wall thickening or mass lesions. The perirectal fat and ischiorectal fossa are unremarkable. The uterus is orthotopic with smooth borders. It displays a normal configuration and appropriate development for age. The myometrium shows homogeneous density. The uterine cavity is normally developed, and the adnexa are unremarkable. The vaginal fornix is normal.

The adequately distended urinary bladder has smooth outer contours and normal wall thickness. The vessels of the lesser pelvis are normal in course and caliber. There are no signs of lymphadenopathy.

The appearance of the pelvic skeleton, especially the femoral heads, sacroiliac joints, and symphysis pubis, is normal. There are no significant soft-tissue abnormalities.

Interpretation

The lesser pelvis appears normal at CT.

Checklist

Pelvic inlet	• Configuration
	• Width
	• Symmetry
	• Iliac wings (shape)
	• Iliopsoas muscles:
	— Size
	— Density
	— Symmetry
Intestinal structures (especially the cecum and rectum)	• Position
	• Wall thickness (when normally distended, see below)
	• No circumscribed wall thickening
	• Well-opacified lumen with no soft-tissue mass
Perirectal fat	• Density (fat attenuation)
	• No infiltration
	• No masses
Ischiorectal fossa	• Bilateral symmetry
	• No masses
	• No lymphadenopathy

Uterus	• Position
	• Size
	• Borders (smooth outer contours)
	• Density (see below)
	• Uterine cavity:
	— Configuration
	— Size
	— Density
	— Contents
Cervix, vagina	• Position
	• Size
	• Borders
Ovaries	• Position
	• Size
	• Density
	• Symmetry
	• No masses of soft-tissue or fluid density
Urinary bladder	• Adequate distention
	• Smooth outer contours
	• Wall thickness (see below)
Vessels	• Caliber
	• Course
	• No significant intimal calcifications
Lymph node stations	• No nodal enlargement (>1 cm)
Pelvic skeleton	• Configuration
	• Margins (cortex smooth and sharp with no discontinuities)
	• Bony structures
	• No circumscribed hypo- or hyperdense areas
	• Femoral heads are rounded and centered in acetabula
	• Sacroiliac joints are smooth and of normal width
	• Symphysis pubis (see below)
Subcutaneous tissue and muscles	• Density
	• Extent
	• Borders
	• Symmetry

Important Data

1 Sacroiliac joint spaces:
- Cartilage thickness 2–5 mm (anterior and inferior: 2–3 mm)

2 Uterus:
- Size (variable): Prepubescent: length up to 3 cm, transverse diameter ca. 1 cm
- Nullipara: length up to 8 cm, transverse diameter ca. 4 cm
- Multipara: length up to 9.5 cm, transverse diameter ca. 5.5 cm
- Postmenopausal: length up to 6 cm, transverse diameter ca. 2 cm
- **a** Transverse diameter of upright uterus (= well-distended bladder) ≤ 5 cm
- **b** Uterine cervix: transverse diameter ≤ 3 cm

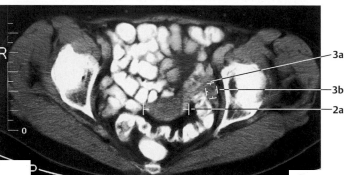

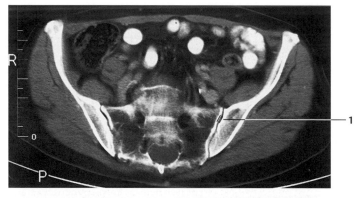

3 **Ovaries:**
- Prepubescence: a, length up to 2.5 cm; b, transverse diameter ca. 2.5 cm
- Sexual maturity: a, length up to 4 cm; b, transverse diameter ca. 2.5 cm
- Postmenopausal: a, length up to 3 cm; b, transverse diameter ca. 1.5 cm

4 **Urinary bladder:**
- Wall thickness (of well-distended bladder): ca. 3 mm

5 **Rectum:**
- Wall thickness ≤ 5 mm

6 **Symphysis pubis:**
- Width < 6 mm

7 **Pelvic dimensions:**
- Pelvic outlet: anteroposterior (= coccyx to posterior edge of symphysis): ca. 9 cm

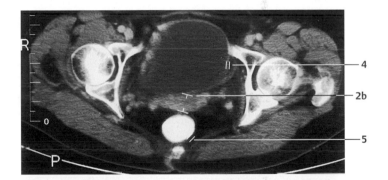

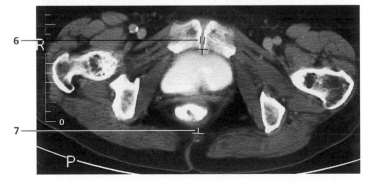

Male Pelvis

The pelvic inlet appears normal, with normal configuration of the iliac wings and iliopsoas muscles.

Imaged bowel structures, especially the cecum and rectum, show no abnormalities with no evidence of wall thickening or mass lesions. The perirectal fat and ischiorectal fossa are unremarkable. The adequately distended urinary bladder has smooth outer contours and normal wall thickness. The seminal vesicles are of normal size. The angle between the bladder and seminal vesicle is clear and normal on each side.

The prostate shows normal size and configuration and a homogeneous internal structure.

The vessels of the lesser pelvis are normal in course and caliber. There are no signs of lymphadenopathy.

The appearance of the pelvic skeleton, especially the femoral heads and sacroiliac joints, is normal.

There are no soft-tissue abnormalities.

Interpretation

The lesser pelvis appears normal at CT.

Checklist

Pelvic inlet	• Configuration
	• Width
	• Symmetry
	• Iliac wings (shape)
	• Iliopsoas muscles:
	— Size
	— Density
	— Symmetry
Intestinal structures (especially the cecum and rectum)	• Position
	• Wall thickness (when normally distended, see below)
	• No circumscribed wall thickening
	• Well-opacified lumen with no soft-tissue mass
Perirectal fat	• Density (fat attenuation)
	• No infiltration
	• No masses
Ischiorectal fossa	• Bilateral symmetry
	• No masses
	• No lymphadenopathy

Urinary bladder	• Adequate distention
	• Smooth outer contours
	• Wall thickness (see below)
Seminal vesicles	• Position (behind the bladder)
	• Size (see below)
	• Symmetry
	• Angle between bladder and seminal vesicle (see below) is clear on each side
Prostate	• Position (central at bladder outlet)
	• Configuration (rounded)
	• Size (see below)
	• Density (homogeneous, see below)
	• No calcifications
	• No unilateral nonhomogeneity after contrast administration
Vessels	• Caliber
	• Course
	• No significant intimal calcifications
Lymph node stations	• No adenopathy
Pelvic skeleton	• Configuration
	• Margins (cortex smooth and sharp, no discontinuities)
	• Bony structures
	• No circumscribed hypodense or hyperdense areas
	• Femoral heads are rounded and centered in acetabula
	• Sacroiliac joints are smooth and of normal width (see below)
	• Symphysis pubis
Subcutaneous tissue and muscles	• Density
	• Extent
	• Borders
	• Symmetry

Important Data

1 Sacroiliac joint spaces:
- Width 2–5 mm (anterior and inferior: 2–3 mm)

2 Urinary bladder:
- Wall thickness (of well-distended bladder): ca. 3 mm

3 Seminal vesicles:
- Size (highly variable):
- **a** Length up to 5 cm
- **b** Width up to 2 cm, height up to 2.5 cm
- **c** Angle between bladder and seminal vesicle: clear on each side

4 Prostate:
- Size (varies with age, 20–70 years):
- **a** Anteroposterior diameter 2.5–3 cm
- **b** Lateral (and craniocaudal diameter) 3–5 cm
- Attenuation value: 40–65 HU

5 Rectum:
- Wall thickness ≤ 5 mm

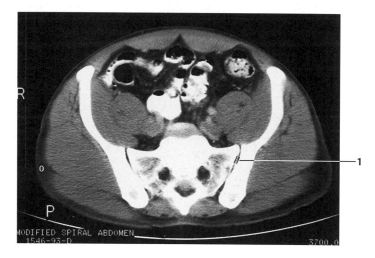

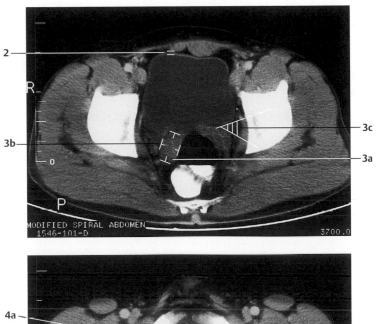

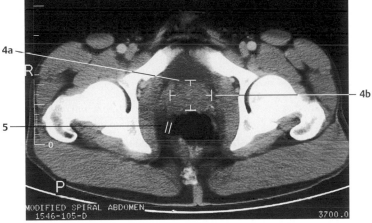

CT: Spinal Column

Cervical Spine

The cervical spine shows a normal degree of lordosis in the lateral survey scan, with no segmental malalignment.

The vertebral bodies show normal configuration and trabecular structure. The cortical margins are of normal thickness and are free of osteophytes.

The bony spinal canal shows normal sagittal diameter.

The intervertebral disks show normal CT density and normal posterior concavity. The disks do not project past the posterior surface of the vertebral bodies. The spinal cord is centrally placed and of normal width. It has homogeneous density and shows no circumscribed narrowing or expansion.

The nerve roots show a normal course and passage through the neuroforamina, which are of normal size and structure. The facet joints and uncovertebral joints are unremarkable.

The prevertebral and paravertebral soft tissues show no abnormalities.

Interpretation

The examined segments of the cervical spine appear normal.

Checklist

Position	• Cervical lordosis
	• No segmental malalignment (lateral survey scan)
	• Normal position of dens (see below)
Bony spinal canal	• Width (see below)
	• Shape
Vertebral bodies	• Shape
	• Cortex (thickness, margins: smooth, sharp)
	• No marginal osteophytes
	• Trabeculae (uniform honeycomb arrangement, no rarefaction or circumscribed voids, no narrowing or expansion)

	• Bony structure (if evaluable: no lytic defects, fracture lines, or osteoplastic areas)
Intervertebral disk space	• Width
	• Margins (smooth, sharp)
	• Straight posterior disk contour
	• No disk protrusion past posterior surface of adjacent vertebral bodies
Spinal cord	• Position (central)
	• Width (see below)
	• No circumscribed narrowing or expansion
	• Density (homogeneous)
	• Perimedullary thecal space clear: — No encroachment from the anterior side (e.g., by an intervertebral disk or osteophyte) or posterior side (e.g., by a hypertrophic ligamentum flavum)
Neuroforamina	• Configuration
	• Width
	• No encroachment from the anterior side (e.g., by an intervertebral disk, osteophyte, or uncovertebral arthrosis) or posterior side (e.g., by hypertrophic spondylarthrosis)
Nerve roots	• Course and passage through the neuroforamina
	• No circumscribed expansion
Facet joints	• Shape, symmetry
	• Pars interarticularis
	• Vertebral arches intact
	• Spinous processes (shape, length, bony structure)
Soft tissues	• Symmetrical arrangement on both sides of the vertebral bodies and spinous processes
	• No masses
	• Prevertebral soft-tissue structures (especially the pharynx and thyroid gland; no masses)

Important Data

1 **Anteroposterior diameter of preodontoid space:**
   - < 2 mm
2 **Sagittal diameter:**
   - C1 ≥ 21 mm
   - C2 ≥ 20 mm
   - C3 ≥ 17 mm
   - C4–C7 = 14 mm

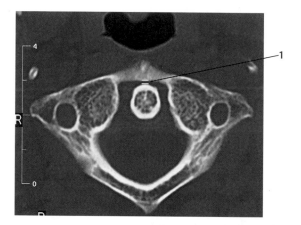

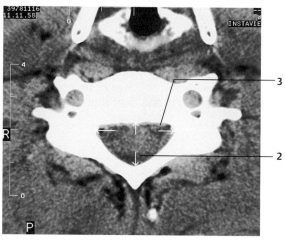

3 Width of spinal canal:
- Transverse diameter at level of pedicles > 20–21 mm

4 Width of spinal cord:
- > 6–7 mm in sagittal plane

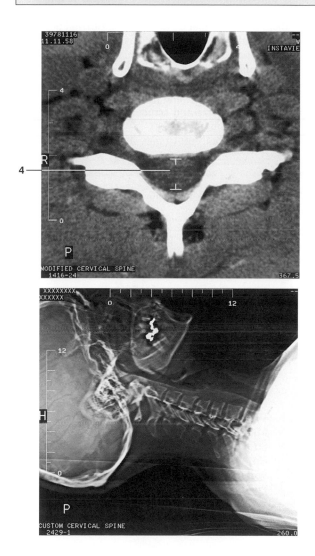

Thoracic Spine

The thoracic spine shows a normal degree of kyphosis in the lateral survey scan, with no segmental malalignment.

The vertebral bodies show normal shape and trabecular structure. The cortical margins are of normal thickness and are free of osteophytes.

The bony spinal canal has normal sagittal diameter.

The intervertebral disks show normal CT density and normal posterior concavity. The disks do not project past the posterior surface of the vertebral bodies. The spinal cord is centrally placed and of normal width. It has homogeneous density and shows no circumscribed narrowing or expansion.

The nerve roots show a normal course and passage through the neuroforamina, which are of normal size and structure. The costovertebral and costotransverse joints are unremarkable.

The prevertebral and paravertebral soft tissues show no abnormalities.

Interpretation

The examined segments of the thoracic spine appear normal.

Checklist

Position	• Thoracic kyphosis
	• No segmental malalignment (lateral survey scan)
Bony spinal canal	• Width (see below)
	• Shape
Vertebral bodies	• Shape
	• Cortex (thickness, margins: smooth, sharp)
	• No marginal osteophytes
	• Trabeculae (uniform honeycomb arrangement, no rarefaction or circumscribed voids, no narrowing or expansion)
Intervertebral disk space	• Width (see below)
	• Margins (smooth, sharp)
	• Straight posterior disk contour
	• No disk protrusion past posterior surface of vertebral bodies
Spinal cord	• Position (central)
	• Width
	• No circumscribed narrowing or expansion
	• Density (homogeneous)

	• Perimedullary thecal space clear: no encroachment from the anterior side (e.g., by an intervertebral disk or osteophyte) or posterior side (e.g., by a hypertrophic ligamentum flavum)
Neuroforamina	• Configuration
	• Width
	• No encroachment from the anterior side (e.g., by an intervertebral disk or osteophyte) or posterior side (e.g., by hypertrophic spondylarthrosis)
Nerve roots	• Course and passage through the neuroforamina
	• No circumscribed expansion
Facet joints	• Shape, symmetry
	• Pars interarticularis
	• Vertebral arches intact
	• Spinous processes (shape, length, bony structure)
	• Costotransverse joints
	• Costovertebral joints (no hypertrophy)
	• Ribs
Soft tissues	• Symmetrical arrangement on both sides of the vertebral bodies and spinous processes
	• No masses
	• Prevertebral soft-tissue structures (especially the lungs, heart, and aorta)

Important Data

1 **Width of spinal canal:**
   - Transverse diameter at level of pedicles > 20–21 mm
2 **Sagittal diameter:**
   - T1–T11 = 13–14 mm, T12 = 15 mm
3 **Jones-Thomson ratio (= A×B/C×D):**
   - Between 0.5 and 0.22 = normal (< 0.22 = spinal stenosis)
4 **Width of intervertebral disk spaces:**
   - Smallest at T1
   - T6–T11: ca. 4–5 mm
   - Largest at T11–T12

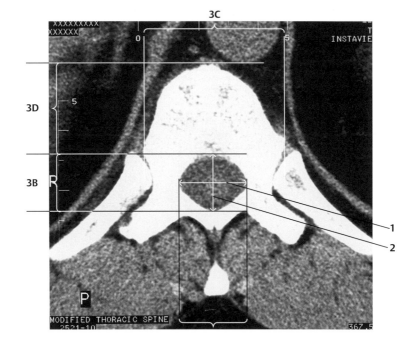

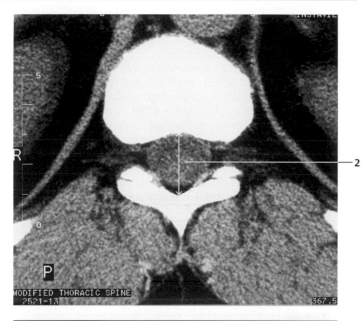

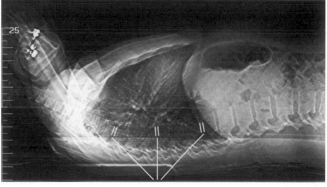

Lumbar Spine

The lumbar spine shows normal lordotic curvature in the lateral survey scan, with no segmental malalignment.

The vertebral bodies have normal shape and trabecular structure. The cortical margins are of normal thickness and are free of osteophytes.

The bony spinal canal has a normal sagittal diameter.

The intervertebral disks show normal density and normal posterior concavity. The disks do not project past the posterior surface of the vertebral bodies.

The conus medullaris shows a normal position at L1 with normal subdivision into filaments. The dural sac is of normal width.

The nerve roots show a normal course and passage through the neuroforamina, which are of normal size and structure. The facet joints are unremarkable.

The prevertebral and paravertebral soft tissues show no abnormalities.

Interpretation

The examined segments of the lumbar spine appear normal.

Checklist

Position	• Lumbar lordosis
	• Lumbosacral angle (see below)
	• No segmental malalignment (lateral survey scan)
Bony spinal canal	• Shape
	• Width (see below)
Vertebral bodies	• Shape
	• Cortex (thickness, margins: smooth, sharp)
	• No marginal osteophytes
	• Trabeculae (uniform honeycomb arrangement, no rarefaction or circumscribed voids, no narrowing or expansion)
Intervertebral disk space	• Width (see below)
	• Margins (smooth, sharp)
	• No disk protrusion past posterior surface of vertebral bodies (posterior disk contour is concave at L1–L4, straight at L4/5, and slightly convex at L5/S1)
Dural tube	• Normal width

	• No circumscribed narrowing or expansion
	• Contents of fluid attenuation
	• Conus medullaris (at L1 level, configuration)
	• Filaments show normal width and arrangement with no posterior adhesion and no circumscribed anterior encroachment (e.g., by an intervertebral disk or osteophyte) or posterior encroachment (e.g., by a hypertrophic ligamentum flavum)
Neuroforamina	• Configuration
	• Width
	• No anterior encroachment (e.g., by an intervertebral disk, osteophyte, or uncovertebral arthrosis) or posterior encroachment (e.g., by hypertrophic spondylarthrosis)
Nerve roots	• Course and passage through the neuroforamina
	• No circumscribed expansion
Facet joints	• Shape, symmetry
	• Pars interarticularis
	• Vertebral arches intact
	• Spinous processes (shape, length, bony structure)
Soft tissues	• Symmetrical arrangement on both sides of the vertebral bodies and spinous processes
	• No masses
	• Prevertebral soft-tissue structures (aorta, vena cava), no masses

Important Data

1 **Lumbosacral angle (S1/horizontal plane):**
   - 26–57°
2 **Width of intervertebral disk space or height of lumbar intervertebral disks:**
   - Approx. 8–12 mm, increasing from L1 to L4/5, decreasing again at L5/S1
3 **Width of spinal canal:**
   - Transverse diameter at level of pedicles: L1–L4 > 20–21 mm, L5 > 24 mm
4 **Sagittal diameter:**
   - 16–18 mm (simple formula: not less than 15 mm; 11–15 mm = relative stenosis, less than 10 mm = absolute stenosis)
5 **Jones-Thomson ratio (= A×B/C×D):**
   - Between 0.5 and 0.22 = normal (<0.22 = spinal stenosis)
6 **Lateral recess (sagittal diameter):**
   - > 4–5 mm
7 **Ligamenta flava:**
   - Width < 6 mm
8 **CT density of intervertebral disks:**
   - 70 ± 5 HU

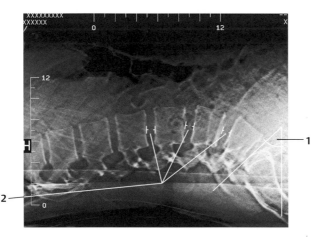

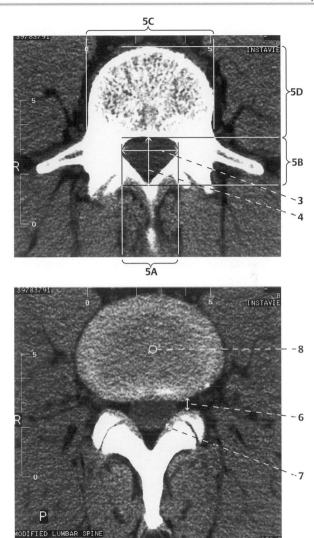

Magnetic Resonance Imaging

MRI: Head and Neck

Neurocranium

The interhemispheric fissure is centered on the midline. The cerebrum and cerebellum exhibit normal cortical sulcation.

The cerebral ventricles are of normal size and symmetrical with normal circulation of CSF. There are no signs of increased intracranial pressure. The cortex and white matter show normal development and normal signal intensity, especially in the periventricular white matter.

No abnormalities are seen in the basal ganglia, internal capsule, corpus callosum, or thalamus.

The brain stem and cerebellum show no abnormal changes in signal characteristics.

The sella and pituitary are normal, and parasellar structures are unremarkable.

The cerebellopontine angle area appears normal on each side. The internal acoustic meatus has normal width.

The paranasal sinuses and mastoid air cells show normal development and pneumatization. The orbital contents are unremarkable.

Interpretation

Cranial MRI is normal.

Checklist

Interhemispheric fissure	• Centered on the midline
	• No displacement
	• Falx cerebri:
	— Width
	— Signal characteristics
	— Flow in the dural sinuses (if the sequence permits flow assessment)
Cortical sulcation in the cerebrum and cerebellum (arbor vitae)	• Configuration
	• Number of sulci
	• Width of sulci
	• No coarsening of sulci

Cerebral cortex	• No circumscribed widening or narrowing
	• Cisterns and cortical markings are well defined
	• Width
	• Distribution (no ectopic tissue)
	• Signal characteristics (no hyperintense [demyelination, edema, hemorrhage] or hypointense [calcification, hemorrhage] changes)
	• No areas of separation from the calvarium
	• No abnormal fluid collection (convex or concave) between the cerebral cortex and calvarium
Ventricles	• Shape
	• Size normal for age (see below)
	• Symmetry (no unilateral or circumscribed enlargement)
	• Evidence of flow in the (centrally located) aqueduct
	• Fourth ventricle is tent-shaped and not dilated
	• No signs of increased intracranial pressure (e.g., effaced sulci, narrowed or widened ventricles)
White matter	• Signal characteristics (maturity appropriate for age; homogeneous signal intensity, especially at periventricular sites; no patchy or circumscribed hyperintense [demyelination, edema, hemorrhage] or hypointense [calcification, hemorrhage] signal changes)
	• Normal width in relation to cortex
Basal ganglia, internal and external capsule, thalamus	• Position
	• Size
	• Delineation
	• Signal intensity
Corpus callosum	• Anatomy
	• Configuration
	• Size
	• No circumscribed narrowing or expansion
	• No foci of demyelination
	• No masses
Brain stem	• Shape
	• Signal intensity (homogeneous)
	• No focal abnormalities
	• Cranial nerves (presence, course, width, symmetry)

Cerebellum	• Anatomy (symmetry) • Cortex (width, sulcation) • White matter (homogeneous signal intensity)
Intracranial vessels	• Course • Width • No abnormal dilatation • No vascular malformations
Sella and pituitary	• Size (see below) • Configuration (surface flat or slightly concave, infundibulum centered) • Signal intensity (neurohypophysis and adenohypophysis, no circumscribed change in signal intensity before or after contrast administration) • Parasellar structures (optic chiasm, suprasellar CSF spaces, carotid siphon, cavernous sinus) are unremarkable

Petrous pyramids	• Cerebellopontine angle area:
	  — Width of internal auditory canals (see below)
	  — CSF spaces (symmetrical, fluid intensity)
	  — No masses
	  — Vestibulocochlear nerve clearly defined
	• Mastoid cells, mastoid antrum
	  — Anatomy
	  — Pneumatization
	  — Borders (wall thickness, smooth and continuous contours)
	  — No masses
	  — Not fluid-filled
	• Cochlea and semicircular canals:
	  — Anatomy
	  — Configuration
	  — Smooth borders

Paranasal sinuses	• Anatomy
	• Pneumatization
	• Borders (wall thickness, smooth and continuous contours)
	• Nasal cavity:
	  — Pneumatization
	  — Septum on midline
	  — Turbinates (presence of superior, middle, and inferior turbinates; width)

Orbit
- Configuration of orbital cone
- Contents:
    - Globe (position, size, signal intensity, wall thickness)
    - Eye muscles (position, course, signal intensity, width)
    - Optic nerve (course, width—see below)
    - Ophthalmic vein (course, width—see below)

Important Data

Vetricular dimensions:
1 **Cella media index:**
   - B/A > 4 = normal
2 **Frontal horn of lateral ventricle (at level of foramen of Monro):**
   - Under 40 years: < 12 mm
   - Over 40 years: < 15 mm
3 **Width of third ventricle:**
   - < 5 mm in children (slightly more in infants)
   - < 7 mm in adults under age 60
   - < 9 mm in adults over age 60

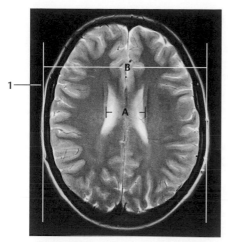

Axial image

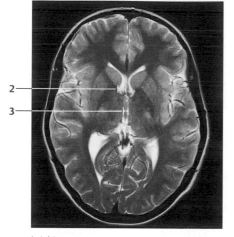

Axial image

4 Width of ophthalmic vein:
- 3–4 mm

5 Optic nerve (axial image):
- **a** Retrobulbar segment: 5.5 mm ± 0.8 mm
- **b** Narrowest point (at approximately mid-orbit): 4.2 mm ± 0.6 mm

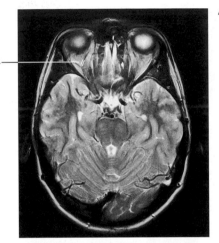

Axial image

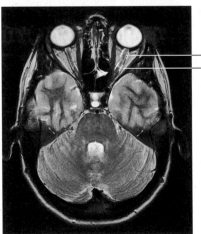

Axial image

6 Position of globe:
- Posterior margin of globe 9.9 mm ± 1.7 mm behind interzygomatic line

7 Internal auditory canal:
- Approximately 5–10 mm, with no more than 1 mm difference between the right and left sides

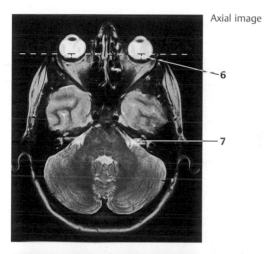

Axial image

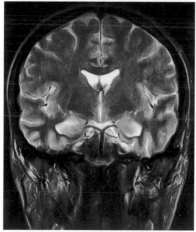

Coronal image

8 Pituitary:
- Height of pituitary in sagittal plane: 2–6 mm

Caution: normal size variations during
— Pregnancy: up to 12 mm
— Puberty: up to 10 mm in girls, up to 8 mm in boys

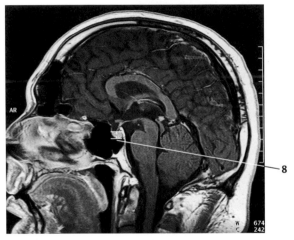

— 8

Sagittal image

Pituitary

The size, position, and configuration of the sella are normal. The floor and walls of the sella are smooth and well-defined.

The pituitary is normal in size, shape, and position. The pituitary tissue shows normal signal characteristics both before and after contrast injection, with no circumscribed abnormalities of signal intensity.

The infundibulum is centered and of normal size.

The optic chiasm and suprasellar CSF spaces appear normal.

The cavernous sinus and imaged portions of the internal carotid artery and carotid siphon are unremarkable.

Evaluable portions of the neurocranium show no abnormalities.

The sphenoid sinus is clear and pneumatized.

Interpretation

The pituitary appears normal.

Checklist

Sella	• Position
	• Size
	• Configuration (U-shaped)
	• Walls steep, not splayed
	• Borders smooth, sharp, and of normal width
Pituitary	• Position (centered in the sella)
	• Configuration (bean-shaped)
	• Superior border straight or slightly concave (convex only during puberty or pregnancy)
	• Size (see below)
	• Delineation of adenohypophysis and neurohypophysis (sagittal image)
	• Pituitary tissue homogeneous on noncontrast images
	• Homogeneous contrast enhancement
	• No circumscribed hypointense or hyperintense areas (especially on coronal images, no signal difference between left and right halves of pituitary)
	• Dynamic sequence (if performed) shows no time differential in the enhancement of different pituitary areas

Infundibulum	• Position (centered)
	• Size (see below)
Optic chiasm	• Position
	• Size (see below)
	• Symmetry
Suprasellar CSF spaces (chiasmatic cistern)	• Symmetrical
	• Not constricted
Cavernous sinuses	• Symmetry
	• Size
	• No infiltration
Internal carotid arteries	• Symmetry
	• Size (especially in siphon area)
	• No circumscribed or generalized narrowing or expansion
Neurocranium	• Temporal lobe
	• Hypothalamus
	• Floor of third ventricle
Sphenoid sinus	• Smooth margins, normal width (especially of the roof), clear and pneumatized

---

Important Data

Pituitary

1 Sagittal diameter:
- Men and postmenopausal women: < 8 mm
- Women of childbearing age: < 10 mm

2 Height in sagittal plane:
- 2–6 mm (*Caution:* normal size variations during
  - Pregnancy: up to 12 mm
  - Puberty: up to 10 mm in girls, up to 8 mm in boys

3 Pituitary stalk:
- < 4 mm

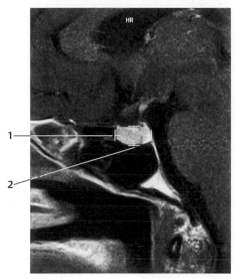

Sagittal image

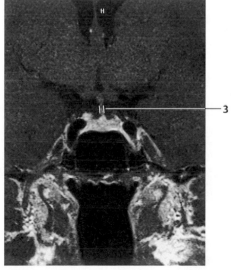

Coronal image

4 Optic chiasm:
- Coronal: **a**, width 9–18 mm; **b**, height 3–6 mm
- Axial: **c**, width 12–27 mm; **d**, depth 4–9 mm

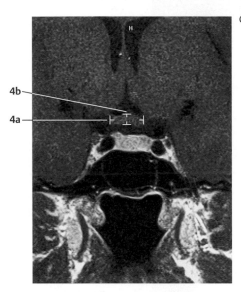

Coronal image

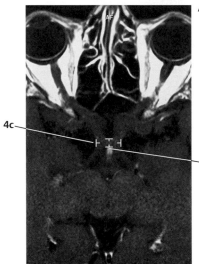

Axial image

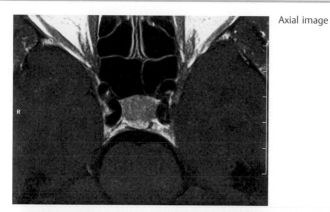

Axial image

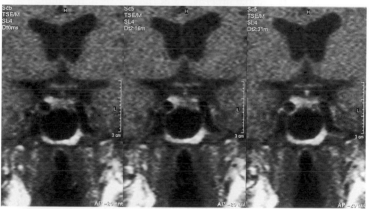

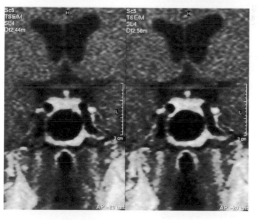

Coronal image: dynamic examination following intravenous contrast administration (Gd-DTPA: gadolinium diethylene-triamine pentaacetic acid)

Internal Auditory Canals, Petrous Pyramids

The petrous pyramids appear normal and symmetrical. The internal acoustic meatus is of normal width, and its walls are smooth and sharply defined. The vestibulocochlear nerve on each side shows normal course and diameter. Contrast administration is not followed by abnormal rise of signal intensity within the nerve, especially its intrameatal portion.

The cochlea and semicircular canals appear normal. The mastoid air cells are clear and pneumatized. The tympanic cavity and external auditory canal are normal.

The cerebellopontine angle area shows normal configuration on each side.

The brain stem shows normal configuration and normal signal characteristics, with normal emergence of the nerves of the auditory canal.

The cerebellopontine angle cistern is clear and symmetrical on each side.

The other imaged portions of the neurocranium are unremarkable.

Interpretation

The internal auditory canals appear normal.

Checklist

Petrous pyramids	• Configuration
	• Bilateral symmetry
	• Internal auditory canals:
	— Shape
	— Course
	— Width (see below)
	— Borders (smooth, sharp)
Vestibulocochlear nerve (cranial nerve VIII)	• Course (straight, continuous)
	• Width (uniform, no right-left discrepancy, no circumscribed expansion)
	• Enhancement characteristics (nonenhancing, especially within the meatus)
Facial nerve (cranial nerve VII)	• Course (starts parallel to vestibulocochlear nerve)
	• Width (uniform, no right-left discrepancy, no circumscribed expansion)
	• Enhancement characteristics (nonenhancing)

Cochlea and semicircular canals	• Anatomy • Configuration • Smooth borders
Mastoid cells, mastoid antrum, tympanic cavity	• Anatomy • Pneumatization • Borders (wall thickness, smooth and continuous contours) • No masses • Not opacified by material of soft-tissue or fluid signal intensity
External auditory canal	• Anatomy • Course • Width • Borders

Cerebellopontine angle area	• Brain stem:
	  — Shape
	  — Signal intensity (homogeneous)
	  — No focal abnormalities
	• Vestibulocochlear and facial nuclei (motor root in medial eminence on floor of fourth ventricle):
	  — No demyelination
	  — No masses
	• Sites of entry of vestibulocochlear nerve (enters pons and medulla at lateral extension of medullopontine sulcus) and facial nerve:
	  — Bilaterally symmetrical
	• CSF spaces:
	  — Cerebellopontine angle cistern (symmetrical, fluid intensity)
	  — No masses
	  — Well delineated
	  — No vascular loops

Rest of neuro-cranium	• Cerebrum (especially the temporal lobe) and cerebellum:
	  — Configuration
	  — Sulcation
	  — Cortical markings (arbor vitae) not effaced
	  — Width of sulci
	  — No circumscribed narrowing or expansion
	  — Homogeneous signal intensity of cortex and white matter (no hypointense or hyperintense changes)

CSF spaces
- Prepontine cistern
- Fourth ventricle

Important Data

1 **Internal auditory canal:**
- Approximately 5–10 mm
2 **Difference between right and left internal auditory canals:**
- Approximately 1 mm

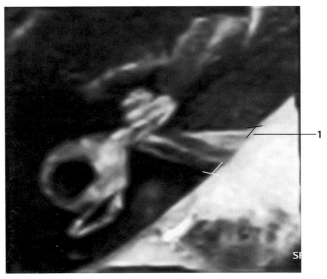

Axial image

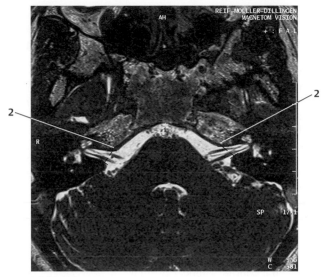

Axial image

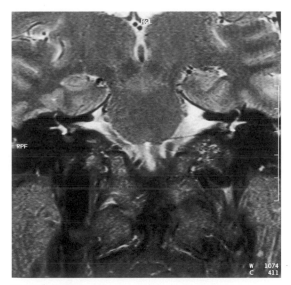

Coronal image

Orbit

The orbits are symmetrical and of normal size, with normal development of the orbital cones. The orbital walls show a normal configuration with smooth, sharp margins. No foci of bone destruction, no circumscribed expansion of the bony or soft-tissue components of the orbital wall are evident.

The globes are symmetrical and of normal size and position, and the ocular contents show normal signal characteristics. The ocular walls are smooth, sharply defined, and of normal thickness. The optic nerve has normal course and caliber on each side.

The eye muscles are normally positioned and display normal course and width. The retrobulbar fat, ophthalmic vein, and lacrimal gland are unremarkable.

Evaluable portions of the neurocranium and paranasal sinuses show no abnormalities.

Interpretation

The orbits and orbital contents appear normal.

Checklist

Orbits	• Shape (orbital cone)
	• Size
	• Symmetry
	• Orbital walls:
	— Borders (smooth and sharp)
	— No bone destruction
	— No circumscribed expansion of bony or soft-tissue components of the orbital wall
Globe	• Shape (spherical)
	• Size (see below)
	• Position (see below)
	• Symmetry
	• Ocular contents:
	— Signal intensity (fluid-equivalent)
	• Ocular wall:
	— Borders (smooth and sharp)
	— Thickness
	• Retrobulbar fat (clear)
	• No masses

Optic nerve	•	Caliber (see below)
	•	Course
Eye muscles	•	Position
	•	Width (see below)
	•	Course
Ophthalmic vein	•	Course
	•	Caliber (see below)
Lacrimal gland	•	Size
	•	Symmetry
	•	No unilateral or bilateral enlargement
	•	Position (see below)
	•	No excavation or destruction of adjacent bone
	•	Homogeneous internal structure
	•	No hypointense or hyperintense changes
	•	Smooth borders
Neurocranium	•	Temporal lobes
	•	Frontal lobes
Paranasal sinuses	•	Maxillary sinuses
	•	Ethmoid cells

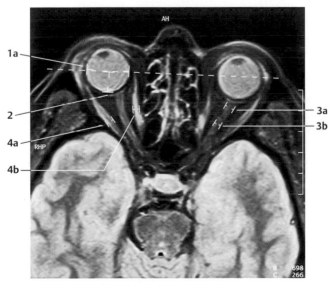

Axial image through center of orbits

Important Data

1 Diameter of globe:
  a Axial image plane: right 28.6 ± 1.2 mm
                       left 29.4 ± 1.4 mm
  b Sagittal image plane: right 27.8 ± 1.2 mm
                          left 28.2 ± 1.2 mm

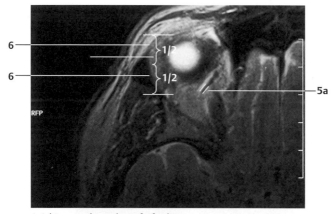

Axial image through roof of orbit

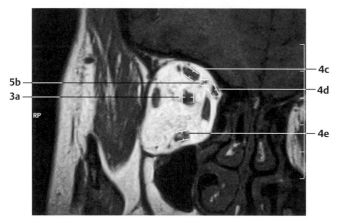

Coronal image

2 Position of globe:
- Posterior margin of globe is 9.9 mm ± 1.7 mm behind interzygomatic line

3 Optic nerve (axial image plane):
- **a** Retrobulbar segment: 5.5 mm ± 0.8 mm
- **b** Narrowest point (at approximately mid-orbit): 4.2 mm ± 0.6 mm

4 Eye muscles:
- **a** Lateral rectus: 2.9 mm ± 0.6 mm
- **b** Medial rectus: 4.1 mm ± 0.5 mm
- **c** Superior rectus: 3.8 mm ± 0.7 mm
- **d** Oblique: 2.4 mm ± 0.4 mm
- **e** Inferior rectus: 4.9 mm ± 0.8 mm
- **f** Levator palpebrae superioris: 1.75 mm ± 0.25 mm

5 Ophthalmic vein:
- **a** 1.8 mm ± 0.5 mm (axial image, 4 mm slice thickness)
- **b** 2.7 mm ± 1 mm (coronal image)

6 Lacrimal gland:
- Less than one-half of the gland is anterior to the frontozygomatic process

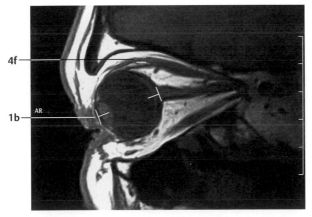

Sagittal image

Paranasal Sinuses

The frontal sinuses are normally developed, clear, and pneumatized with smooth wall contours.

The ethmoid cells show normal development and intact bony walls, with no defects on the orbital side. There are no areas of wall erosion or mucosal thickening.

The sphenoid sinus is normally developed and presents a coarse honeycomb structure. There are no fluid collections or mucosal swelling.

The maxillary sinuses are bilaterally symmetrical and have smooth walls of normal thickness. The sinuses are clear and aerated with no foci of bone erosion or destruction. The nasal septum is centered on the midline. The nasal turbinates show a normal arrangement and normal signal intensity.

The nasal cavity, pharynx, and imaged parapharyngeal structures show no abnormalities.

Interpretation

The paranasal sinuses appear normal.

Checklist

Frontal sinuses	• Anatomy
	• Wall contours (smooth)
	• Pneumatization
Ethmoid cells	• Anatomy
	• Pneumatization
	• Bony structures (especially bordering the orbit: contours are smooth, sharp, and intact)
	• No wall erosion
	• No mucosal thickening
Sphenoid sinus	• Anatomy (coarse honeycomb structure)
	• Clear and pneumatized
	• No fluid collection
	• No mucosal swelling
	• Bony structures (smooth, intact walls, no erosion)
	• No extrinsic wall indentations
Maxillary sinuses	• Anatomy
	• Size (bilaterally symmetrical)
	• Bony structures (smooth, intact contours, normal wall thickness, no bone erosion or destruction)

Nasal cavity	• Pneumatization
	• No tooth roots projecting through sinus floor
	• Anatomy (symmetry)
	• Size
	• Aeration (clear)
	• Septum centered on the midline
	• Nasal turbinates (three per side: superior, middle, inferior) are normally developed
	• Signal characteristics
Pharynx and parapharyngeal structures	• Anatomy (symmetry)
	• Size
	• Wall thickness
	• No foreign bodies
	• No masses
Neurocranium (especially the temporal and frontal lobes)	• Cortex
	• White matter
	• Gyration
	• Signal characteristics
Orbit	• Eye muscles (width, signal characteristics)
	• Optic nerve (width, course)
	• Globe (shape, size, signal characteristics)
	• Retrobulbar fat (no masses)

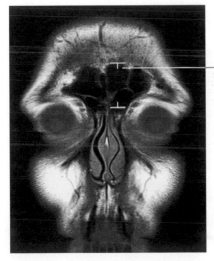

Coronal image

Important Data

1 **Frontal sinus:**
   • Height ca. 1.5–2 cm
2 **Sphenoid sinus:**
   • Width 0.9–1.4 cm
3 **Maxillary sinuses;**
   a Width ca. 2 cm
   b Height ca. 2 cm

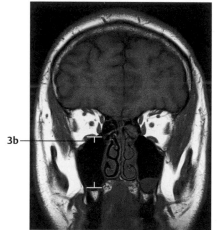

Coronal image

3b

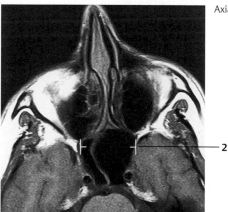

Axial image

2

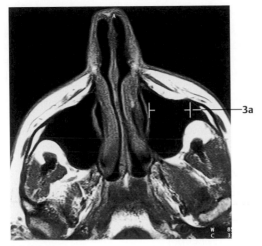

Axial image

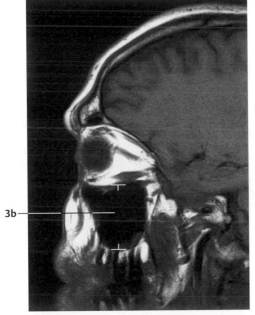

Sagittal image

Cervical Soft Tissues

The cervical soft tissues show normal configuration. The position of the cervical spine is normal.

The oral floor muscles are normally developed and bilaterally symmetrical. The spaces of the oral cavity and neck are clear and well defined.

Imaged portions of the parotid and submandibular glands show no abnormalities.

The pharynx and larynx show normal boundaries and normal wall thickness.

The thyroid gland shows reasonable symmetry and normal size. The thyroid lobes display normal internal structure.

Cervical vessels that are evaluable with MRI have normal appearance. The muscular structures of the neck are normal.

There are no signs of cervical lymphadenopathy.

No abnormalities are seen in the cervical spinal cord or cervical plexus.

Interpretation

The cervical soft tissues appear normal.

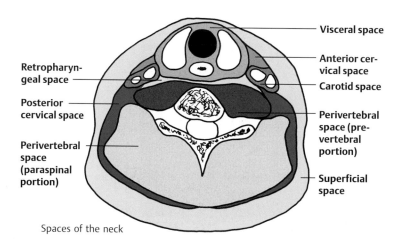

Spaces of the neck

Checklist

Cervical soft tissues	• Configuration • Normal anatomy • Normal position of the cervical spine (see below)
Oral floor muscles	• Anatomy • Width • Bilateral symmetry • Delineation • Internal structure • Spaces of oral floor are clearly defined
Submandibular and parotid glands	• Size (symmetry) • Signal characteristics • No dilatation of glandular duct • No hypointense or hyperintense areas within the glandular tissue
Pharynx and larynx	• Shape (symmetrical) • Size • Smooth walls • Normal wall thickness • No masses

Cervical spaces	• Retropharyngeal space
	• Parapharyngeal space (visceral space)
	• Carotid space
	• Anterior and posterior cervical spaces
	• Perivertebral space (prevertebral and paraspinal portions):
	  — Configuration
	  — Borders
	  — Symmetry
	  — Internal structure
	  — Width (see below)

Esophagus	• Position • Wall thickness (see below) • Borders • No masses
Thyroid gland	• Anatomy (consists of two lobes, reasonably symmetrical) • Size (see below) • Internal structure (homogeneous) • No cysts • No nodules

Cervical vessels	• Course
	• Caliber (see below)
	• No abrupt caliber changes
Neck muscles	• Anatomy
	• Symmetry
	• Borders
	• Signal characteristics (internal structure)
Lymph node stations (if evaluable)	• No lymphadenopathy
Cervical spine (if evaluable)	• Vertebral bodies
	— Number
	— Shape
	— Position
	— Contours
	• Bone marrow signal
	• Intervertebral disk spaces
	• Spinal canal:
	— Width
	— No circumscribed narrowing
	• Normal width of cervical spinal cord
	• No masses
	• No narrowing
Cervical plexus	• No appreciable narrowing
	• No masses (including lymphadenopathy)

Important Data

Ch = Chamberlain's line (line connecting the posterior part of the hard palate with the posterior rim of the foramen magnum):
- Tip of the dens projects no more than 1 ± 6.6 mm past Chamberlain's line

Prevertebral soft tissues:
1. Retropharyngeal:
   - Approximately 1.7 ± 0.7 mm
2. Retroglottic:
   - Approximately 6.0 ± 1.1 mm
3. Retrotracheal:
   - Approximatley 8.4 ± 2.5 mm

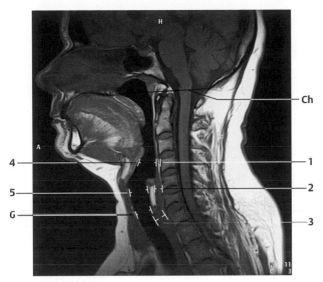

Midsagittal image

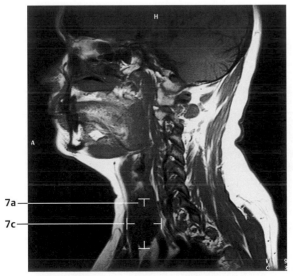

Sagittal image

Lumina of upper respiratory tract (normal respiration):
4 Laryngeal inlet (hyoid level):
  - Approximatley 19 ± 4 mm
5 Glottis:
  - Approximately 21 ± 4 mm
6 Trachea:
  - Approximately 17 ± 3 mm
7 Dimensions of thyroid gland:
  a Length: 3.5–6 cm
  b Width: 1.5–2 cm
  c Depth: 1–2 cm
Vascular calibers (at level of thyroid gland):
8 Common carotid artery:
  - 6–10 mm
9 Esophagus:
  - Wall thickness 3 mm

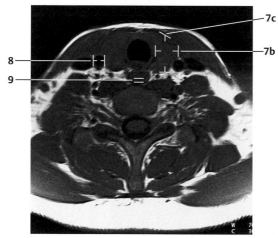

Axial image

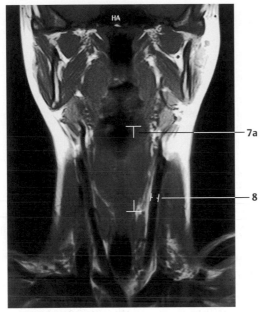

— 7a

— 8

Coronal image

MRI: Chest

Thoracic Organs

Both lungs are normally aerated and are applied to the chest wall on all sides. The pleurae show normal homogeneous signal intensity, and there are no fluid collections.

The pulmonary structure is normal and presents normal vascular markings. There are no intrapulmonary nodules or patchy densities.

The mediastinum is centered and of normal width. There is no evidence of masses in the anterior, central, or posterior compartment.

The hilar region on each side is unremarkable, and the main bronchi appear normal. There is no lymphadenopathy and there are no perihilar masses.

The heart is orthotopic and has a normal configuration. The cardiac chambers are of normal size.

Major intrathoracic vessels are unremarkable, and imaged portions of the supra-aortic vessels appear normal.

The thoracic skeleton and thoracic soft tissues show no abnormalities.

Interpretation

The thoracic organs appear normal.

Checklist

Lungs	• Anatomy (paired and symmetrical)
	• Fully apposed to the chest wall
	• No pleural thickening
	• No fluid collection (patchy or circumscribed)
	• Normal aeration
	• Normal low signal of the lung parenchyma
	• Normal pulmonary structure
	• Vascular markings diminish from center to periphery
	• No pulmonary nodules
	• No larger densities (e.g., plaques or infiltrates)
Mediastinum	• Configuration
	• Position:

- — Centered
- — Width (see below)
- — No masses in the anterior, central, or posterior compartment
- Hilar region:
  - — No masses
  - — No lymphadenopathy
- Main bronchi:
  - — Anatomy
  - — Course
  - — Width (see below)
- Heart:
  - — Position (centered slightly left of midline)
  - — Configuration
  - — Size of cardiac chambers (see below)
  - — Normal myocardial thickness (see below)

Vessels
- Intrathoracic vessels (ascending aorta, aortic arch, descending aorta, vena cava):
  - — Anatomy
  - — Size
- Supra-aortic vessels (subclavian artery, brachiocephalic trunk, left common carotid artery):
  - — Anatomy
  - — Size

Diaphragm
- Shape (bell-shaped, no contour abnormalities, costophrenic angle is sharp and clear)
- Position (at approximately the level of the 10th–11th posterior rib)
- Width (no circumscribed widening, no defect)

Thoracic skeleton (ribs, clavicle, sternum, scapula)
- Position
- Structure and signal characteristics
- Contours and symmetry
- No bony expansion or destruction
- Thoracic spine:
  - — Position and shape of thoracic vertebrae
  - — Spinal cord
  - — Signal characteristics of thoracic vertebrae

Thoracic soft tissues
- Normal
- Symmetrical

Important Data

1 **Angle of tracheal bifurcation:**
- Approximately 55–65°

2 **Diameter of main bronchi:**
  a Right approx. 15 mm
  b Left approx. 13 mm

3 **Diameter of aorta:**
- < 4 cm
  a Ascending aorta:
    a_1 At level of pulmonary trunk bifurcation: 3.2 cm ± 0.5 cm
    a_2 At level of aortic root: 3.7 cm ± 0.3 cm
  b Aortic arch: 1.5 cm ± 1.2 cm
  c Descending aorta: 2.5 cm ± 0.4 cm
Ratio of ascending to descending aortic diameters = 1.5:1

4 **Diameter of superior vena cava:**
  a At level of aortic arch: 1.4 cm ± 0.4 cm
  b At level of pulmonary trunk bifurcation: 2 cm ± 0.4 cm

5 **Diameter of pulmonary arteries:**
  a Pulmonary trunk: 2.4 cm ± 0.2 cm
  b Proximal right pulmonary artery: 1.9 cm ± 0.3 cm
  c Left pulmonary artery: 2.1 cm ± 0.4 cm

6 **Mediastinum:**
- Thymus 1–2 cm in transverse diameter

Heart:

Dimensions of cardiac chambers:

7 **Right atrium:**
- Maximum transverse diameter: 4.4 cm
  a At level of aortic root: 1.9 cm ± 0.8 cm
  b At level of mitral valve: 3.2 cm ± 1.2 cm
  c At center of ventricles: 2.8 cm ± 0.4 cm

8 **Left atrium:**
  a Maximum anteroposterior diameter: 4–5 cm
    a_1 At level of aortic root: 2.4 cm ± 4.5 cm
    a_2 At level of mitral valve: 2.9 cm ± 4.9 cm
  b Maximum transverse diameter: 9 cm
    b_1 At level of aortic root: 5.5 cm ± 8.4 cm
    b_2 At level of mitral valve: 4.9 cm ± 9.1 cm

9 **Angle between midsagittal plane and septum** = 38° (increases in response to pressure loading or volume loading of the ventricles)

10 **Thickness of ventricular septum:**
- Approximately 5–10 mm

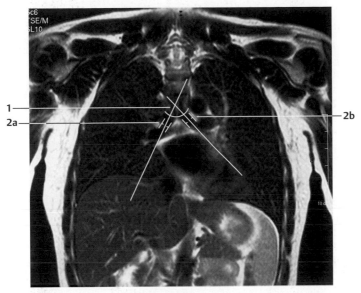

Coronal image

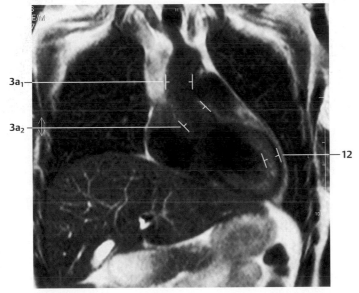

Coronal image

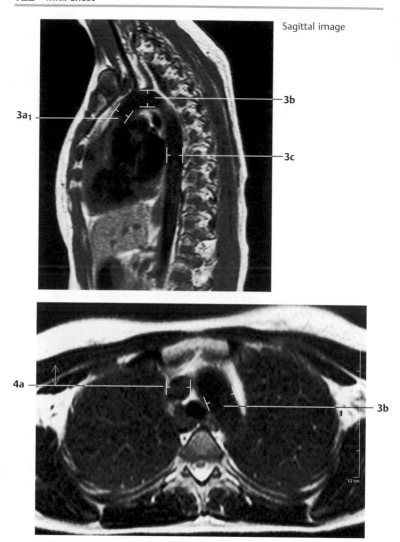

Sagittal image

Axial image at level of aortic arch

---

11 Thickness of pericardium:
- 1–2 mm

12 Thickness of myocardium:
- 10–12 mm

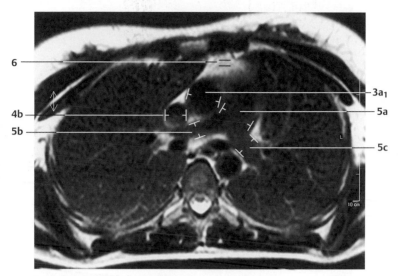

Axial image at level of pulmonary trunk bifurcation

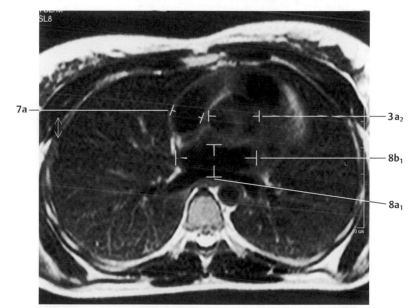

Axial image at level of aortic root

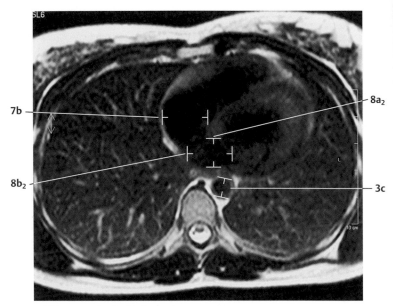

Axial image at level of mitral valve

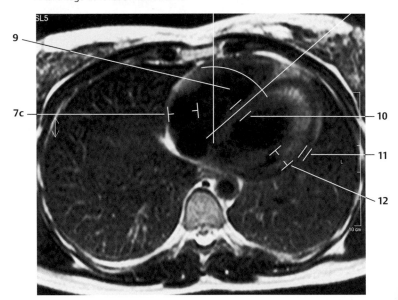

Axial image through center of ventricles

Breast

The anatomy of the glandular breast tissue is symmetrical and normal for age. The breast parenchyma is uniformly subdivided by fatty tissue. Unenhanced MR images show no lesions that are hypointense or hyperintense to the breast parenchyma or fat.

Following contrast administration, a significant, abnormal rise in signal intensity is not observed in any segment of the breast.

The skin and subcutaneous tissues show no abnormalities.

Interpretation

The breasts appear normal.

Checklist

Breast parenchyma	• Size
	• Symmetry
	• Extent of breast parenchyma in relation to fat (note physiological involution of the parenchyma with aging)
	• Symmetrical development of glandular breast tissue
	• Uniform subdivision by fat
Noncontrast images	• No lesions that are hypointense or hyperintense to the breast parenchyma or fat (cysts, solid tumors, stellate densities)
Postcontrast images	• No significant abnormal enhancement (more than about 70% of initial signal intensity in the early phase after contrast administration)
	• No abnormal enhancing structures on delayed images
	• Early, intense enhancement of the nipple area (confirms proper injection technique)
Skin and subcutaneous tissues	• Thickness
	• No retraction
	• No circumscribed expansion
Axilla (unless obscured by motion artifacts)	• No lymphadenopathy

Lungs (unless obscured by motion artifacts)
- Complete aeration
- No pulmonary nodules
- Bony structures (ribs and sternum, unless obscured by motion artifacts):
  — Contours
  — Shape
  — No voids or expansion
  — Retrosternal structures (lymph nodes along internal thoracic artery) appear grossly normal

Heart (unless obscured by motion artifacts)
- Shape
- Size
- Position
- Enhancement characteristics

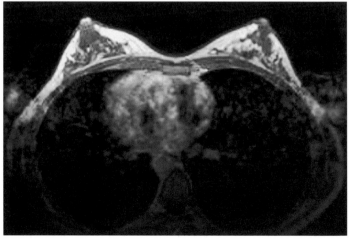

Axial image through the center of the breasts following contrast administration (Gd DTPA: gadolinium diethylenetriaminepentaacetate)

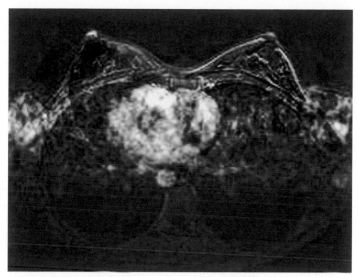

Subtraction image of the breasts

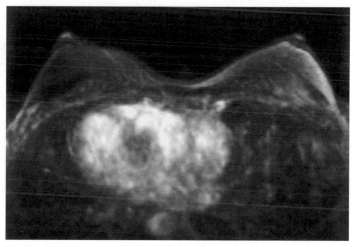

3-D MIP (Maximum Intensity Projection) rendering of subtraction images

MRI: Abdomen

Upper Abdominal Organs

The liver is normally positioned and has normal size and smooth borders. Its internal structure is normal, with no focal abnormalities of signal intensity. The intrahepatic and extrahepatic bile ducts are not distended. The porta hepatis appears normal.

The gallbladder displays a normal size, smooth borders, and homogeneous contents.

The spleen is orthotopic and of normal size. It has smooth outer contours and a homogeneous internal structure.

The pancreas is normal in size and position. The head, body, and tail of the organ have smooth, lobulated outer contours and normal internal structure. The pancreatic duct is unobstructed.

Both kidneys are normal in size and position. The renal parenchyma shows normal width and structure.

The renal pelvis and calices are normal. The urinary drainage tract is unobstructed.

Both adrenal glands are normal in position and size, and the adrenal crura are normally developed. The adrenal compartment is unremarkable.

Major vessels and the para-aortic region appear normal, with no evidence of lymphadenopathy.

Imaged portions of the lung and soft tissues show no abnormalities.

Interpretation

The upper abdominal organs appear normal.

Checklist

Liver
- Position
  - Directly below the right hemidiaphragm
- Size (see below)
- Borders:
  - Smooth
  - Sharp
- No focal abnormalities
- Intrahepatic bile ducts:
  - Course (toward porta hepatis)
  - Width
  - No calculi
  - No air
- Extrahepatic bile ducts:
  - Course (from porta hepatis to head of pancreas)
  - Width (see below)
  - Homogeneous contents of fluid-equivalent signal intensity
  - No calculi
  - No air
- Gallbladder:
  - Size (see below)
  - Contours (smooth)
  - Wall thickness (see below)
  - No pericholecystic fluid
- Gallbladder contents:
  - Homogeneous
  - Fluid-equivalent signal intensity
  - No calculi (hypointense or hyperintense)
  - No air
- Porta hepatis occupied by the hepatic artery, common bile duct, and portal vein
- No masses
- No lymphadenopathy

Spleen
- Size (see below)
- Smooth outer contours
- Homogeneous internal structure

Pancreas
- Size normal for age (see below)
- Normal lobulation
- Smooth outer contours

	• Pancreatic duct unobstructed (see below)
	• No peripancreatic fluid
Kidneys	• Paired
	• Position (see below)
	• Size (see below)
	• Smooth contours
	• Width of cortex and medulla
	• Renal pelvis (presence, symmetry, size, no widening, homogeneous fluid contents)
	• Calices (shape, width, homogeneous contents)
	• Enhancement characteristics (see below)
Ureters	• Not duplicated
	• Course
	• No obstruction of urinary drainage
Adrenal glands	• Shape
	• Size (see below)
	• Slender crura (no asymmetric widening)
	• No circumscribed hypointense (T1: cyst, adenoma), isointense, or hyperintense expansion
Intestinal structures	• Colon haustrations
	• Small bowel
	• Wall thickness
	• Homogeneous opacification with oral contrast medium (if administered)
	• No free extraintestinal or intra-abdominal air or fluid
	• Para-aortic region:
	— Major vessels (position, size, fluid signal)
	— Soft tissues (no masses)
	— No lymphadenopathy
Lungs	• Clear and expanded
Costophrenic sinus	• Clear and aerated on both sides
Soft tissues	

Important Data

Dimensions

1 Liver:

  a Left lobe (anteroposterior diameter on the left paravertebral line): up to 5 cm

  b Caudate lobe/right lobe (CL/RL) = 0.37 ± 0.16 (e.g., 0.88 ± 0.2 in cirrhosis). Reference lines [from medial side]: line I is tangent to the medial border of the caudate lobe; line II is parallel to I and tangent to the lateral aspect of the portal vein; line III is tangent to the lateral hepatic border and perpendicular to a line midway between the portal vein and inferior vena cava and perpendicular to I and II.

  c Angle of hepatic border: ca. 45° on the left side (formed by left lateral and inferior hepatic borders)

2 Gallbladder:

  a Horizontal diameter up to 5 cm (> 5 cm is suspicious for hydrops)

  b Width of gallbladder wall: 1–3 mm

3 Width of common bile duct:

  • ≤ 8 mm (≤ 10 mm after cholecystectomy)

4 Spleen:

  a Depth: 4–6 cm

  b Width: 7–10 cm

  c Length: 11–15 cm

  Splenic index: D × W × L = 160–440

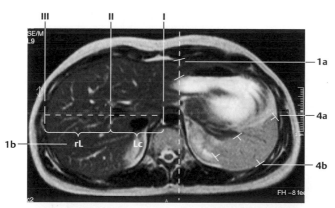

Axial image

5 **Pancreas:**
   a Head: up to 3.5 cm
   b Body: up to 2.5 cm
   c Tail: up to 2.5 cm
   Pancreatic duct: width 1–3 mm
6 **Adrenal glands (variable):**
   • Crural thickness < 10 mm
7 **Kidneys:**
   a Craniocaudal diameter: 8–13 cm
   b Anteroposterior diameter: ca. 4 cm
   c Transverse diameter 5–6 cm
   Position of superior poles of kidneys:
   d Right: superior border of L1
   d Left: inferior border of T12
   f Transverse renal axis: posteriorly divergent angle of 120°
   g Width of renal cortex: 4–5 mm
   Time to corticomedullary equilibrium: 1 minute
   Contrast excretion into the pyelocaliceal system: 3 minutes
   Gerota fascia (thickness): 1–2 mm
   Width of ureter: 4–7 mm
8 **Diameter of abdominal aorta:**
   • Approximately 18–30 mm
9 **Inferior vena cava:**
   • Transverse diameter up to 2.5 cm
Lymph nodes larger than 1 cm are suspicious for pathology.

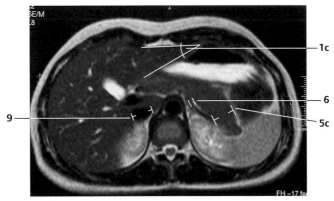

Axial image

2b
5a
2a
5b
3
8

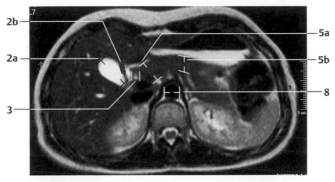

Axial image

7f
7b
7g
7c

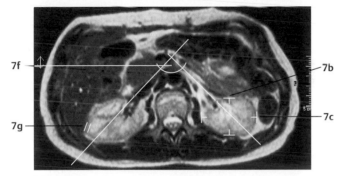

Axial image

7e
4c
7d
7a
7a

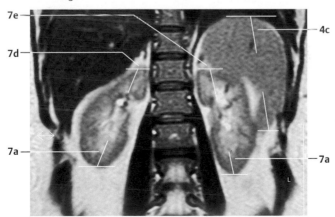

Coronal image

Liver

The liver is orthotopic and presents normal size and smooth borders. It has a normal internal structure with no focal abnormalities. The intrahepatic and extrahepatic bile ducts are not dilated.

The gallbladder appears normal, displaying smooth borders and homogeneous contents.

The porta hepatis shows no abnormalities.

Other visualized upper abdominal organs are unremarkable.

Interpretation

The liver appears normal.

Checklist

Liver

- Position
  - Directly below the right hemidiaphragm
- Size (see below)
- Borders:
  - Smooth
  - Sharp
- No focal abnormalities
- Intrahepatic bile ducts:
  - Course (toward porta hepatis)
  - Width
  - No calculi
  - No air
- Extrahepatic bile ducts:
  - Course (from porta hepatis to head of pancreas)
  - Width (see below)
  - Homogeneous contents of fluid-equivalent signal intensity
  - No calculi
  - No air

- Gallbladder:
  - Size (see below)
  - Contours (smooth and sharp)
  - Wall thickness (see below, no general or circumscribed thickening)
  - No pericholecystic fluid
- Gallbladder contents:
  - Homogeneous
  - Fluid-equivalent signal intensity
  - No filling defects (calculi, polyps)
  - No air
- Porta hepatis:
  - Occupied by the hepatic artery, common bile duct, and portal vein
  - No masses
  - No lymphadenopathy
- Costophrenic sinus is clear and aerated on each side

Spleen
- Normal size (see below)
- Homogeneous internal structure

Pancreas
- Normal size (see below)
- Pancreatic duct unobstructed (see below)

Para-aortic region
- Unremarkable

Kidneys (if visualized)
- Position
- Size
- Internal structure

Intestinal structures
- Normal
- No free extraintestinal or intra-abdominal air or fluid

Important Data

Dimensions:

1 Liver:

  a Left lobe (anteroposterior diameter on the left paravertebral line): up to 5 cm

  b Right lobe (craniocaudal diameter measured on the midclavicular line): up to ca. 15 cm

  Angle of hepatic border:

  c Right side: ca. 75° (inferior border, sagittal plane)

  d Left side: ca. 45° (left lateral and inferior borders)

  e Caudate lobe/right lobe (CL/RL) = 0.37 ± 0.16 (e.g., 0.88 ± 0.2 in cirrhosis). Reference lines [from medial side]: line I is tangent to the medial border of the caudate lobe; line II is parallel to I and tangent to the lateral aspect of the portal vein; line III is tangent to the lateral hepatic border and perpendicular to a line midway between the portal vein and inferior vena cava and perpendicular to I and II.

2 Gallbladder:

  a Horizontal diameter up to 5 cm (> 5 cm is suspicious for hydrops)

  b Width of gallbladder wall: 1–3 mm

3 Width of common bile duct:

  • ≤ 8 mm (after cholecystectomy: ≤ 10 mm)

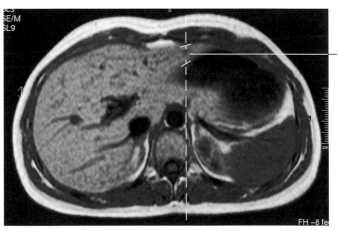

T1-weighted noncontrast axial image

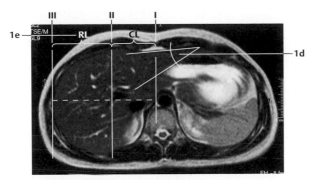

T2-weighted noncontrast axial image

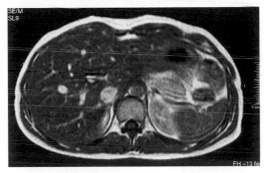

T1-weighted axial image after the i. v. administration of a
superparamagnetic contrast agent

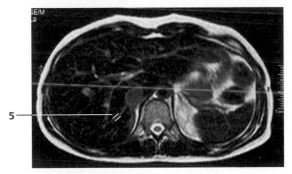

T2-weighted axial image after the i. v. administration of a
superparamagnetic contrast agent

4 Portal vein:
- Up to 1.5 cm

5 Hepatic veins:
- Up to 0.5 cm

Spleen:
- Depth D): 4–6 cm
- Widt(W): 7–10 cm
- Length (L): 11–15 cm
- Splenic index: DxWxL = between 160 and 440

Adrenal glands (variable):
- Crural thickness < 10 mm

Kidneys:
- Craniocaudal diameter: 8–13 cm
- Anteroposterior diameter: ca. 4 cm
- Transverse diameter: 5–6 cm

Position of superior poles of kidneys:
- Right: superior border of L1; left: inferior border of T12

Transverse renal axis:
- Posteriorly divergent angle of 120°

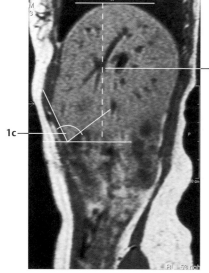

Sagittal image at the level of the mid-clavicular line

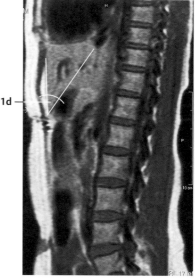

Sagittal image through the left lobe of the liver

Width of renal cortex:
- 4–5 mm

Diameter of abdominal aorta:
- Approximately 18–30 mm

Inferior vena cava:
- Transverse diameter: up to 2.5 cm

Lymph nodes larger than 1 cm are suspicious for pathology.

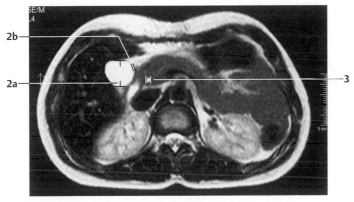

Axial image

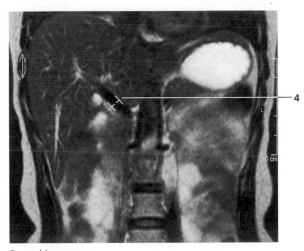

Coronal image

Kidneys

Both kidneys appear normal in size and position, and the renal parenchyma displays normal width. There is no evidence of a mass.
The calices are of normal shape, and the renal pelvis appears normal. The urinary drainage tract is unobstructed.
Postcontrast images show a normal time to corticomedullary equilibrium and undelayed, symmetrical contrast excretion into the renal pelves.
Other visualized upper abdominal organs, especially the adrenal glands, show no abnormalities.

Interpretation

Both kidneys appear normal.

Checklist

Kidneys
- Paired
- Position (see below)
- Size (see below)
- Contours:
  - Smooth
- Parenchymal width and signal (see below)
- Normal relation of cortex to medulla
- Renal pelves:
  - Structure
  - Bilateral symmetry
  - Width
  - Shape of calices
- Ureters:
  - One per side
  - Course
  - Width (see below)
  - No obstruction of urinary drainage
- Perirenal and pararenal spaces:
  - Fat signal
- Perirenal and pararenal fasciae:
  - Position
  - Width (no circumscribed thickening)

Adrenal glands	• Shape
	• Size (see below)
	• Slender crura
	• No circumscribed expansion
Retroperitoneal space	• No abnormalities (mass, fluid)
Intestinal structures (colon haustrations, small bowel)	• Normal
	• Wall thickness
	• No free extraintestinal or intra-abdominal air or fluid
Major vessels	• Course
	• Caliber (see below)
	• No lymphadenopathy (see below)
Soft tissues	• Fat signal
	• Bilateral symmetry

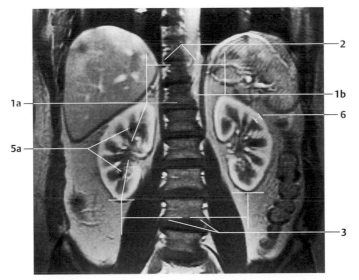

T1-weighted coronal image using breath-hold technique, early bolus phase

Important Data

1 **Position of superior poles of kidneys:**
   a Right: superior border of L1
   b Left: inferior border of T12 (variable; right kidney is lower than left kidney by up to one vertebral body height)

2 **Distance between superior renal poles:**
   • Approximately 10 cm (4–16 cm)

3 **Distance between inferior renal poles:**
   • Approx. 13 cm (9–18.5 cm)

4 **Transverse renal axis:**
   • Posteriorly divergent angle of 120°

5 **Renal dimensions:**
   • Craniocaudal 8–13 cm (<1.5 cm craniocaudal difference in renal sizes)
   Transverse renal diameter at level of hilum: 5–6 cm (b = transverse) × 3–4 cm (c = anteroposterior)

6 **Renal cortical thickness:**
   • 4–5 mm

7 **Time to corticomedullary equilibrium:**
   • 1 minute

8 **Contrast excretion into the pyelocaliceal system:**
   • 3 minutes

9 **Width of ureter:**
   • 4–7 mm

10 **Gerota fascia (thickness):**
   • 1–2 mm

11 **Abdominal aorta:**
   • Transverse diameter ca. 18–30 mm

12 **Inferior vena cava:**
   • Transverse diameter up to 2.5 cm
   Lymph nodes larger than 1 cm are suspicious for pathology.

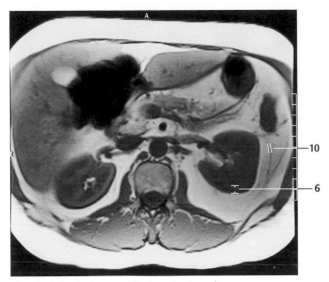

T1-weighted axial image without contrast medium

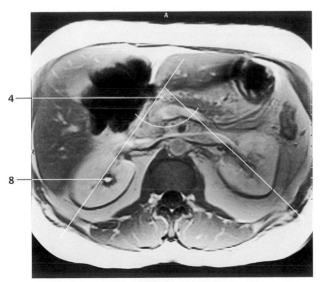

T1-weighted axial image after contrast administration

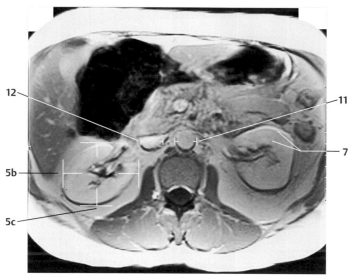

T1-weighted axial image after contrast administration

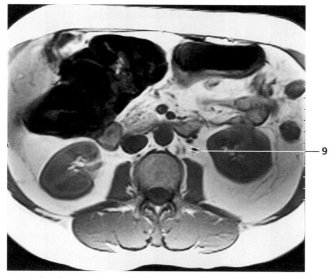

T1-weighted noncontrast axial image at the level of the ureters

Adrenal Glands

Both adrenal glands present normal size and position with normally developed crura. There is no evidence of a mass or circumscribed expansion.

The adrenal compartment appears normal.

Postcontrast images show normal adrenal enhancement characteristics and dynamics.

No abnormalities are found in other visualized upper abdominal organs, especially the kidneys.

Interpretation

Both adrenal glands appear normal.

Checklist

Adrenal glands
- Paired
- Position (superior and anterior to kidneys)
- Shape, size (see below)
- Borders (smooth, sharp)
- Signal characteristics of normal adrenals (T1: slightly hypointense to liver; T1 fat-saturated: isointense; T2: hypointense; T2 fat-saturated: hyperintense)
- No circumscribed hypointense, isointense or hyperintense expansion of adrenal crura (e.g., T2-weighted signal is increased in many pheochromocytomas) or circumscribed hypointense or hyperintense lesions (e.g., calcifications, fat deposits)
- Enhancement characteristics:
  - Adenomas show moderate signal increase that usually returns to initial level by 10 minutes postinjection
  - Most malignant tumors still show intense enhancement after 15 minuntes
- Chemical shift imaging:
  - In-phase and out-of-phase T1-weighted images show fat intensity (decreased signal) in benign disease

	• Adrenal compartment:
	  — Fat intensity
	  — No masses

Liver	• Size (see below)
	• Borders:
	  — Smooth
	  — Sharp
	• Homogeneous internal parenchymal structure
	• Intrahepatic and extrahepatic bile ducts
	• Costophrenic sinus is clear and aerated on each side

Spleen	• Size (see below) • Smooth outer contours • Homogeneous internal structure
Pancreas	• Size • Pancreatic duct
Kidneys	• Paired • Position (see below) • Size (see below) • Smooth contours
Stomach and bowel	• Position • Size • No masses • No infiltration
Major blood vessels	• Transverse diameter (see below) • Flow
Lymph nodes **Soft tissues**	• No lymphadenopathy

Important Data

Dimensions:
1 Adrenal glands (variable):
• Crural thickness < 10 mm
Kidneys:
Position of superior poles of kidneys:
• Right: superior border of L1
• Left: inferior border of T12
Transverse renal axis:
• Posteriorly divergent angle of 120°

Thickness of renal cortex:
- 4–5 mm

Renal dimensions:
- Craniocaudal diameter: 8–13 cm
- Anteroposterior diameter: ca. 4 cm
- Transverse diameter: 5–6 cm

Gerota fascia (thickness):
- 1–2 mm

Spleen:
- Width: 7–10 cm
- Depth: 4–6 cm
- Length: 11–15 cm

Diameter of abdominal aorta:
- Approximately 18–30 mm

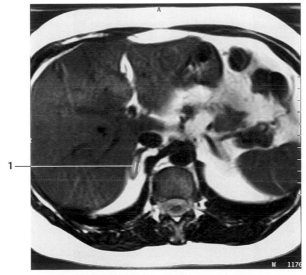

T2-weighted axial image through the adrenal glands

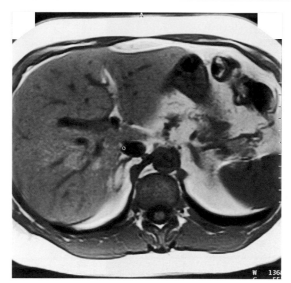

T1-weighted axial image, noncontrast and in-phase

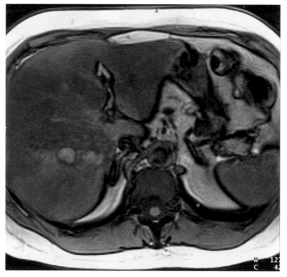

T1-weighted axial image, noncontrast and out-of-phase

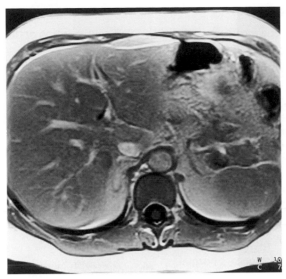

T1-weighted axial image, postcontrast and in-phase

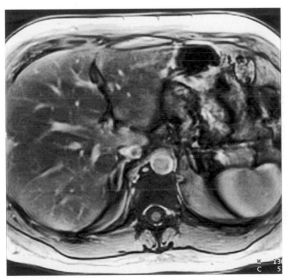

T1-weighted axial image, postcontrast and out-of-phase

Female Pelvis

The pelvic inlet appears normal, with normal configuration of the iliac wings and iliopsoas muscles.

No abnormalities are found in imaged bowel structures, and there are no signs of wall thickening or mass lesions.

The uterus is anteverted and has normal internal structure. The adnexa appear normal on both sides.

The adequately distended urinary bladder appears normal and has a normal wall thickness.

The vessels of the lesser pelvis are normal in course and caliber. There is no apparent lymphadenopathy.

The femoral heads are normally shaped and articulate normally with the acetabula. They have normal bone-marrow signal characteristics.

The soft tissues show no abnormalities.

Interpretation

The lesser pelvis appears normal.

Checklist

Pelvic inlet	• Configuration
	• Width
	• Symmetry
	• Iliac wings (shape)
Iliopsoas muscles	• Size
	• Signal characteristics
	• Symmetry
Intestinal structures (especially the cecum and rectum)	• Position
	• Wall thickness (if with normal distension, see below)
	• No circumscribed wall thickening
	• Well-opacified lumen with no soft-tissue mass
Perirectal fat	• Signal characteristics (fat intensity)
	• No infiltration
	• No masses
Ischiorectal fossa	• Bilateral symmetry
	• No masses
	• No lymphadenopathy
Uterus	• Position
	• Size (see below)
	• Borders (smooth outer contours)

	• Signal characteristics
	• Uterine cavity:
	— Configuration
	— Size
	— Signal characteristics
Cervix, vagina	• Position
	• Size
	• Borders
Ovaries	• Position
	• Size (see below)
	• Signal characteristics
	• Symmetry
	• No masses of soft tissue or fluid signal intensity
Urinary bladder	• Adequate distention
	• Outer contours:
	— Smooth
	— Wall thickness (see below)
Vessels	• Caliber (see below)
	• Course
	• No significant intimal calcifications
Lymph node stations	• No lymphadenopathy
Pelvic skeleton	• Configuration
	• Margins (cortex smooth and sharp, no discontinuities)
	• Fat-equivalent signal intensity of bone marrow
	• No circumscribed areas of marrow replacement
	• Femoral heads rounded and centered in acetabula
	• Sacroiliac joints:
	— Smooth contours
	— Normal width (see below)
	• Symphysis pubis (see below)
Subcutaneous tissue and muscles	• Signal characteristics
	• Extent
	• Borders
	• Symmetry

Important Data

Pelvic dimensions:
1 **True conjugate:**
   - Approximately 11 cm
2 **Pelvic cavity:**
   - > 12 cm
3 **Pelvic outlet:**
   - Approximately 9 cm
4 **Transverse diameter (transverse interspinous distance):**
   - Approximately 13 cm
5 **Uterus (variable):**
   - Prepubescent: **a**, length up to 3 cm; **b**, transverse diameter ca. 1 cm
   - Nullipara: **a**, length up to 8 cm; **b**, transverse diameter ca. 4 cm
   - Multipara: **a**, length up to 9.5 cm; **b**, transverse diameter ca. 5.5 cm
   - Postmenopausal: **a**, length up to 6 cm; **b**, transverse diameter ca. 2 cm
   (Transverse diameter of upright uterus = well distended bladder ≤ 5 cm)
6 **Uterine cervix:**
   a Craniocaudal ≤ 2 cm
   b Transverse diameter ≤ 3 cm

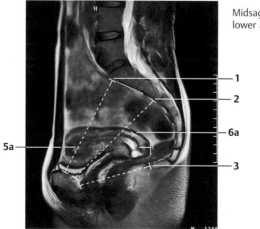

Midsagittal image through the lower abdomen.

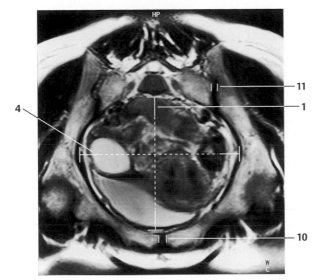

Paracoronal image along the true conjugate (line 1 in Fig. on left [= midsagittal section through the lower abdomen]).

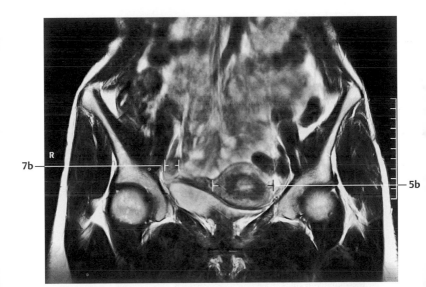

Coronal image

7 **Ovaries:**
- Prepubescent: **a**, length up to 2.5 cm; **b**, transverse diameter ca. 2.5 cm
- Sexual maturity: **a**, length up to 4 cm; **b**, transverse diameter ca. 2.5 cm
- Postmenopausal: **a**, length up to 3 cm; **b**, transverse diameter ca. 1.5 cm

8 **Urinary bladder (well distended):**
- Wall thickness ca. 3 cm

9 **Rectum:**
- Wall thickness ≤ 5 mm

10 **Symphysis pubis:**
- Width < 6 mm

11 **Cartilage thickness of sacroiliac joint spaces:**
- 2–5 mm (anterior and inferior: 2–3 mm)

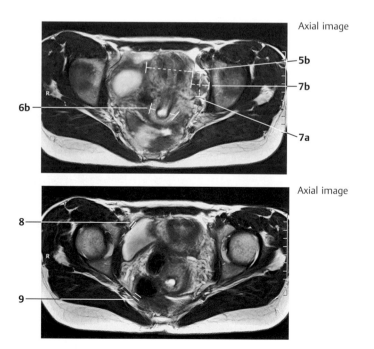

Axial image

Axial image

Male Pelvis

The pelvic inlet appears normal, with normal configuration of the iliac wings and iliopsoas muscles.

No abnormalities are found in imaged bowel structures, and there are no signs of wall thickening or mass lesions.

The distended urinary bladder appears normal and has normal wall thickness. The seminal vesicles are of normal size. The angle between the bladder and seminal vesicle is normal on each side. The prostate shows a normal size and configuration.

The vessels of the lesser pelvis are normal in their course and caliber. There is no evidence of lymphadenopathy.

The femoral heads are normally shaped and articulate normally with the acetabula. They have normal bone-marrow signal characteristics. The soft tissues show no abnormalities.

Interpretation

The lesser pelvis appears normal.

Checklist

Pelvic inlet	• Configuration
	• Width
	• Symmetry
	• Iliac wings (shape)
	• Iliopsoas muscles:
	— Size
	— Signal characteristics
	— Symmetry
Intestinal structures (especially the cecum and rectum)	• Borders
	• Position
	• Wall thickness (if with normal distension, see below)
	• No circumscribed wall thickening
	• Well-opacified lumen with no soft-tissue mass
Perirectal fat	• Signal characteristics (fat intensity)
	• No infiltration
	• No masses
Ischiorectal fossa	• Bilateral symmetry
	• No masses
	• No lymphadenopathy
Seminal vesicles	• Position (behind the bladder)
	• Size (see below)

	• Symmetry
	• Angle between the bladder and seminal vesicle (see below) is clear on each side
	• Signal characteristics
Prostate	• Position (central at bladder outlet)
	• Configuration (rounded shape, intact capsule and lobulation)
	• Size (see below)
	• Homogeneous signal intensity
	• No calcifications
	• No unilateral nonhomogeneity after contrast administration
Urinary bladder	• Adequate distension
	• Smooth outer contours
	• Wall thickness (see below)
Vessels	• Caliber (see below)
	• Course
Lymph node stations	• No lymphadenopathy
Pelvic skeleton	• Configuration
	• Margins (cortex smooth and sharp, no discontinuities)
	• Fat-equivalent signal intensity of bone marrow
	• No circumscribed areas of marrow replacement
	• Femoral heads rounded and centered in acetabula
	• Sacroiliac joints:
	— Smooth contours
	— Width (see below)
	• Symphysis pubis
Subcutaneous tissue and muscles	• Density
	• Extent
	• Borders
	• Symmetry

Important Data

1 Prostate (size varies with age, 20–70 years):
  a Anteroposterior diameter ca. 2.5–3 cm
  b Lateral diameter: 3–5 cm
  c Craniocaudal diameter: 3–5 cm

2 Symphysis pubis:
  • Width < 6 mm

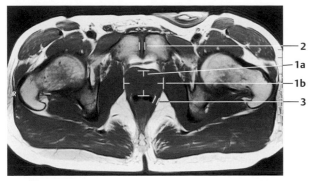

Axial image

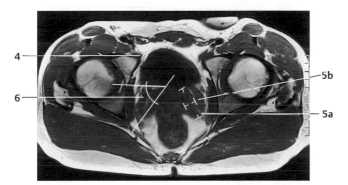

Axial image

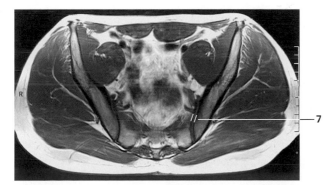

Axial image

3 **Rectum:**
- Wall thickness ≤ 5 mm
4 **Urinary bladder (well distended):**
- Wall thickness ca. 3 mm
5 **Seminal vesicles (highly variable):**
  a Length: up to 5 cm
  b Width: up to 2 cm
6 **Angle between bladder and seminal vesicles:**
- Open = normal
7 **Width of sacroiliac joint spaces:**
- 2–5 mm (anterior and inferior: 2–3 mm)

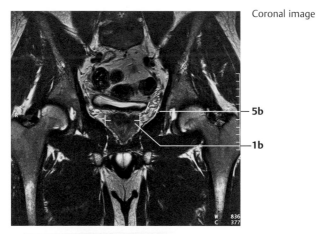

Coronal image

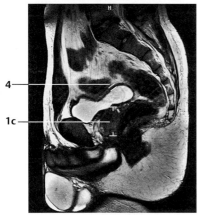

Midsagittal image

Testes

The scrotum and its contents display normal configuration.
The testes are symmetrical and of normal size with a homogeneous internal structure. Each testis is sharply demarcated by the tunica albuginea, which is of normal thickness.
The epididymis shows a normal size and position on each side and presents a normal internal structure.
The scrotal compartments appear normal on each side, with no sign of increased fluid.
The inguinal canal is normal in its shape, size, and course.
The corpora cavernosa and corpus spongiosum are normal.

Interpretation

The testes appear normal.

Checklist

Scrotum	• Size
	• Configuration
Testes	• Paired
	• Symmetrical
	• Size (see below)
	• Homogeneous internal structure (high T2-weighted signal intensity)
	• No circumscribed or diffuse change in signal intensity
Tunica albuginea	• Smooth, sharp borders on all sides
	• Normal thickness
Epididymis (head and tail)	• Position
	• Size (bilateral symmetry)
	• Internal structure
	• Scrotal compartments have smooth, sharp borders
	• No increased fluid
Inguinal canal	• Shape
	• Size
	• Course
Corpora cavernosa	• Size
	• Bilateral symmetry
	• Honeycomb internal structure
Corpus spongiosum	• Size
	• Urethra

Important Data

Testicular dimensions:
1 **Length:**
   • Up to ca. 4 cm
2 **Transverse diameter:**
   • Up to ca. 3 cm

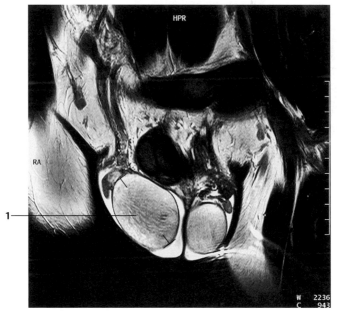

T2-weighted coronal image

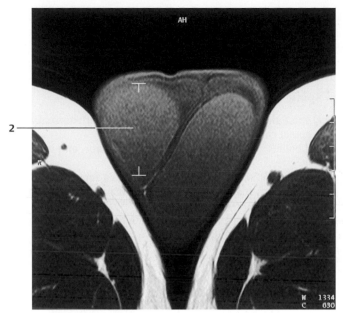

2

T1-weighted axial image

MRI: Spinal Column

Cervical Spine

The cervical spine shows a normal degree of lordosis with normal width of the bony spinal canal.

The vertebral bodies are normal in their number, shape, and interrelationships.

The atlantodental distance is normal. The articulating vertebral end plates present smooth margins. The intervertebral disk spaces are of normal height.

The intervertebral disks do not project past the posterior surface of the vertebral bodies in any imaged segment.

The spinal cord, including the craniocervical junction, displays normal position, configuration, width, and internal structure. The bone marrow of the vertebral bodies appears normal.

The prevertebral and paravertebral soft tissues show no abnormalities.

Interpretation

The cervical spine appears normal.

Checklist

Position	• Normal cervical lordosis (no hypolordosis or hyperlordosis, no kyphotic deformity) • No segmental malalignment • Normal position of the dens (see below)
Bony spinal canal	• Width (see below) • Smooth margins

Vertebral bodies	• Number (seven)
	• Shape (square except for the dens)
	• Position (straight alignment of posterior margins, no steps)
	• End plates
	  — Continuous margins (no discontinuities)
	  — Smooth contours
	  — No circumscribed depression
	  — No marginal osteophytes

Intervertebral disk space	• Width (see below) • Normal signal characteristics: moderate to slightly hyperintense T2-weighted intensity (not hypointense to other disks) • No disk protrusion past posterior surface of adjacent vertebral bodies
Spinal cord	• Configuration • Width • Signal characteristics • No circumscribed change in signal intensity • No circumscribed narrowing or expansion

Nerve roots	• Course
	• Passage through the neuroforamina
	• Dural tube:
	  — Shape
	  — Width
	  — No circumscribed narrowing or expansion
	  — Perimedullary contents of fluid signal intensity

Neuroforamina	• Configuration • Width • No hypertrophy of uncovertebral joints
Facet joints	• Shape • Position • Contours (smooth, continuous) • No hypertrophy • Vertebral arches intact • No shortening of pedicles
Spinous processes	• Shape • Position • Size • Bony structure • Fat-equivalent signal intensity of bone marrow • No circumscribed hypointense or hyperintense areas
Soft tissues	• Symmetrically arranged on both sides of the vertebral bodies and spinous processes • No masses • Prevertebral soft-tissue structures (especially the pharynx and thyroid gland; no masses)

Important Data

1 **Atlantodental distance:**
   a Sagittal plane: approx. 1–3 mm (up to 5 mm in children)
   b Coronal and axial planes: dens is centered
2 **Craniovertebral angle (angle formed by the basilar line and the posterior tangent to C2):**
   - Normal range of 150° (flexion) to 180° (extension) (spinal compression occurs at less than 150°)
3 **Chamberlain's line (line connecting the posterior border of the hard palate with the posterior rim of the foramen magnum):**
   - Tip of the dens should project no more than 1 mm ± 6.6 mm above the line
4 **Retropharyngeal space:**
   - Up to 7 mm (at level of C2)
5 **Width of spinal cord:**
   - Sagittal > 6–7 mm
6 **Sagittal diameter:**
   - C1 ≥ 21 mm
   - C2 ≥ 20 mm
   - C3 ≥ 17 mm
   - C4–C7 = 14 mm
7 **Height of intervertebral disk spaces:**
   - C2 < C3 < C4 < C5 < C6 ≥ C7
8 **Retrotracheal space:**
   - Up to 22 mm (at level of C6)
9 **Anteroposterior diameter of preodontoid space:**
   - < 2 mm
10 **Width of spinal canal:**
   - Transverse diameter at level of pedicles > 20–21 mm

1a —

4 —

7 —

— 3

— 5

— 6

— 8

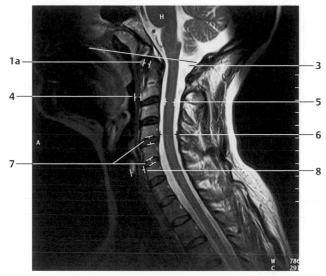

T2-weighted midsagittal image

2 —

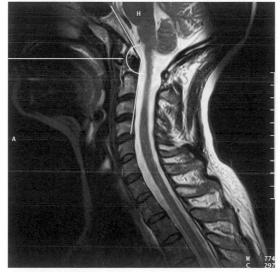

T2-weighted sagittal image

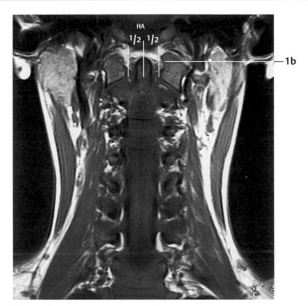

Coronal image

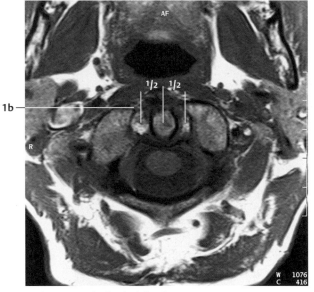

Axial image at the level of the dens

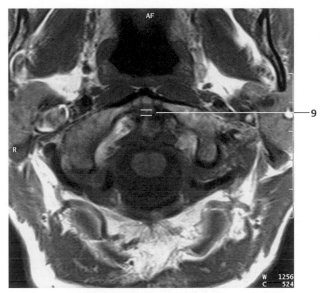

Axial image at the level of the dens

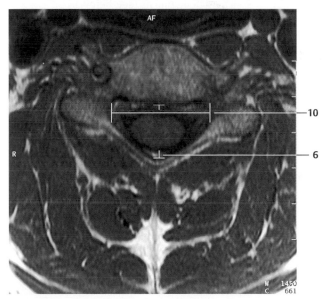

Axial image at the level of the laminae

Thoracic Spine

The thoracic spine shows a normal degree of kyphosis with a normal width of the bony spinal canal.

The vertebral bodies are normal in their number, shape, and interrelationships. The articulating vertebral end plates present smooth margins. The intervertebral disk spaces are of normal height, and the disks do not project past the posterior surface of the vertebral bodies in any segment.

The spinal cord displays normal course, configuration, width, and internal structure.

The bone marrow of the vertebral bodies appears normal.

The prevertebral and paravertebral soft tissues show no abnormalities.

Interpretation

The thoracic spine appears normal.

Checklist

Position	• Thoracic kyphosis (see below)
	• No segmental malalignment
Bony spinal canal	• Width (see below)
	• Smooth margins
Vertebral bodies	• Number (12)
	• Shape (square)
	• Position (straight alignment of posterior margins, no step)
	• End plates
	— Continuous margins
	— No circumscribed depression
	— Smooth contours, no marginal osteophytes
Intervertebral disk space	• Width (see below)
	• Normal signal characteristics: moderate to slightly hyperintense T2-weighted signal intensity (not hypointense to other disks); "nuclear cleft" signifies an adult disk
	• No disk protrusion past posterior surface of adjacent vertebral bodies
Spinal cord	• Configuration
	• Width
	• Signal characteristics

	• No circumscribed signal changes
	• No circumscribed narrowing or expansion
Nerve roots	• Course
	• Passage through the neuroforamina
Dural sack	• Shape
	• Width
	• No circumscribed narrowing or expansion
	• Contents of fluid intensity
Neuroforamina	• Configuration
	• Width
Facet joints	• Shape
	• Position
	• Contours (smooth, continuous)
	• No hypertrophy
	• Vertebral arches intact
	• Pars interarticularis intact
	• No cleft anomalies
	• No shortening of pedicles
Spinous processes	• Shape
	• Position
	• Size
	• Bony structure
	• Fat-equivalent signal intensity of bone marrow
	• No circumscribed hypointense or hyperintense areas
Soft tissues	• Symmetrically arranged on both sides of the vertebral bodies and spinous processes
	• No masses
Aorta	• Prevertebral soft-tissue structures

Important Data

1 **Kyphotic angle (of Stagnara):**
- Angle formed by a line parallel to the vertebral end plates of T3 and T11 = 25°

Width of spinal canal:

2 **Transverse diameter at level of pedicles:**
- > 20–21 mm

3 **Sagittal diameter:**
- T1–T11 = 13–14 mm
- T12 = 15 mm

4 **Width of intervertebral disk spaces:**
- Smallest at T1
- T6–T11: ca. 4–5 mm
- Largest at T11–T12

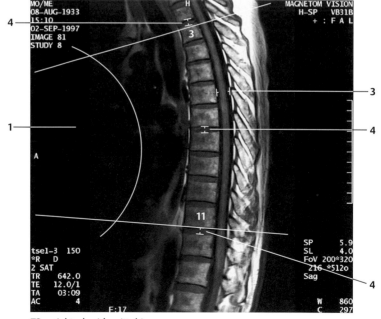

T2-weighted midsagittal image

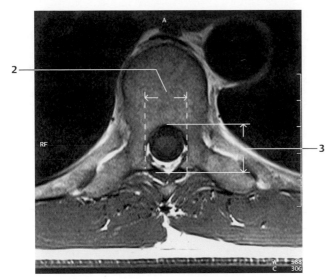

Axial image at the level of the laminae

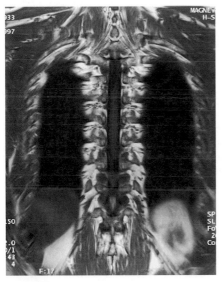

Coronal image

Lumbar Spine

The lumbar spine shows a smooth lordotic curve with a normal promontory angle. The bony spinal canal displays normal width.

The vertebral bodies are normal in their number, shape, and interrelationships. The articulating vertebral end plates present smooth margins. The intervertebral disk spaces are of normal height, and the disks do not project past the posterior surface of the vertebral bodies in any segment.

The conus medullaris terminates normally at the L1 level and divides into its filaments.

The dural tube appears normal in its lumbar portion and evaluable sacral portion.

The bone marrow of the vertebral bodies appears normal.

The imaged soft tissues show no abnormalities.

Interpretation

The lumbar spine appears normal.

Checklist

Position	• Lumbar lordosis (see below)
	• Lumbosacral angle (see below)
	• No segmental malalignment
Bony spinal canal	• Width (see below)
	• Smooth margins
Vertebral bodies	• Number (five)
	• Shape (square)
	• Position (straight alignment of posterior margins, no step)
	• End plates
	— Continuous margins
	— No circumscribed depression
	— Smooth contours
	— No marginal osteophytes
Intervertebral disk space	• Width (see below)
	• Normal signal characteristics: moderate to slightly hyperintense T2-weighted signal intensity (not hypointense to other disks); "nuclear cleft" signifies an adult disk

- No disk protrusion past posterior surface of adjacent vertebral bodies (posterior disk contours on axial images: concave at L1–L4, straight at L4/5, slightly convex at L5/S1)

Conus medullaris
- Configuration
- Width
- No circumscribed narrowing or expansion
- Position (terminates at approximately the L1 level)
- Normal division into filaments
- Signal characteristics
- Filaments:
  — Course (sweeping, not straight; no posterior adhesions)
  — Width
  — No circumscribed mass

Nerve roots
- Course
- Passage through neuroforamina
- Dural sac:
  — Shape
  — Width
  — No circumscribed narrowing or expansion
  — Contents of fluid intensity

Bony portions of vertebral bodies
- Neuroforamina:
  — Configuration
  — Width
- Facet joints:
  — Shape
  — Position
  — Contours (smooth, continuous)
  — No hypertrophy of facet joints
- Vertebral arches intact
- Pars interarticularis intact
- No cleft anomalies
  — No shortening of pedicles
  — Spinous processes:
  — Shape
  — Position
  — Size
  — Bony structure
- Fat-equivalent signal intensity of bone marrow
  — No circumscribed hypointense or hyperintense areas

Soft tissues
- Symmetrically arranged on both sides of the vertebral bodies and spinous processes
- Prevertebral soft-tissue structures
- No masses

Aorta, iliac vessels

Important Data

1 **Width of intervertebral disk space and height of lumbar intervertebral disks:**
- 8–12 mm
- Increases from L1 to L4/5
- Usually decreases at L5/S1, but may be the same as or greater than L4/5

2 **Lordosis (static axis):**
- Plumb line from center of L3 should intersect S1

3 **Lumbosacral angle (S1/horizontal plane)** = 26–57°

4 **Width of spinal canal: sagittal diameter:**
- 16–18 mm (simple formula: not less than 15 mm; 11–15 mm = relative stenosis, less than 10 mm = absolute stenosis)

5 **Width of spinal canal: transverse diameter (at level of pedicles):**
- L1–L4: > 20–21 mm
- L5: > 24 mm

6 **Jones-Thomson ratio (= A × B/C × D):**
- Between 1/2 and 1/4.5 = normal (denominator > 4.5 = spinal stenosis)

7 **Lateral recess (sagittal diameter):**
- > 4–5 mm

8 **Ligamenta flava:**
- Width < 6 mm

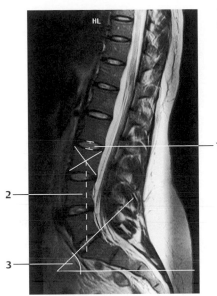

T2-weighted sagittal image at level of lateral recess

1

2

3

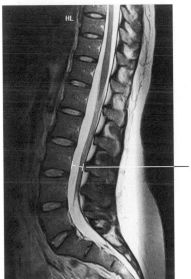

T2-weighted midsagittal image

4

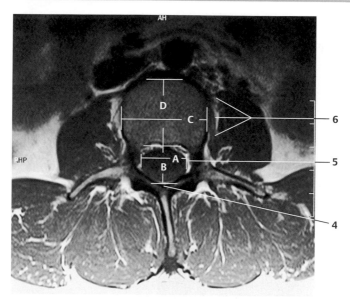

T2-weighted axial image at level of pars interarticularis

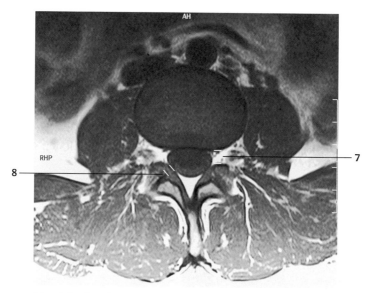

T1-weighted axial image at level of neuroforamina

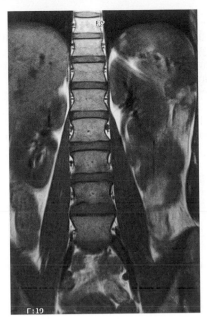

Coronal image

Sacroiliac Joints

The sacroiliac joints are normally shaped with normal development of the sacrum and iliac wings and a normal-appearing lumbosacral junction. The joint space is of normal width on both sides. The joint contours are smooth and sharply defined.

The subchondral bone marrow appears normal. There are no marginal osteophytes.

The sacrum and iliac wings also contain normal bone marrow and present smooth, intact cortical boundaries. The sacral neuroforamina are of normal width.

The nerve filaments shows a normal course and diameter, and the width of the sacral spinal canal is normal.

The muscles and the imaged organs of the lesser pelvis show no abnormalities.

Interpretation

The sacroiliac joints appear normal.

Checklist

Joint
- Shape:
  - Articular surfaces converge posteriorly
  - Bilateral symmetry
- Contours:
  - Margins: smooth, sharp
  - Cortical thickness (uniform)
  - No steps or discontinuities
  - No marginal osteophytes
- Joint space:
  - Uniform normal width (see below)
  - No circumscribed narrowing or expansion
  - No obliteration (ankylosis)
  - No unilateral increase in joint fluid
  - No signal voids within the joint space (air, calcifications)
  - No marginal osteophytes (caution: the ileum normally contains areas of hyperostosis)
  - Normal thickness of articular cartilage (see below)
  - No abnormal contrast enhancement
  - No thickening of joint capsule

- Subchondral region:
  - Homogeneous, fat-equivalent signal intensity of bone marrow
  - No erosive or destructive changes
  - No increase in T2-weighted signal intensity (e.g., circumscribed due to cysts or patchy due to bone-marrow edema)
  - No decrease in T1-weighted or T2-weighted signal intensity (e.g., sclerosis on the sacral side or fatty infiltration of the periarticular bone marrow)

Sacrum
- Anatomy (four vertebral bodies, four neuroforamina)
- Shape
- Symmetry (lateral sacral mass)
- Width and arrangement of neuroforamina
- Bone marrow signal (fat-equivalent, no marrow-replacing process)
- Bony spinal canal (width)
- Shape (closed)
- Dural tube (width, no circumscribed narrowing or expansion)
- Filaments have normal size and arrangement, and are not fused together; no posterior adhesions
- Sacral plexus (course, width)

Iliac wings
- Shape
- Symmetry
- Margins: smooth, sharp
- Cortical thickness (continuous and uniform; no steps or discontinuities)
- Bone marrow signal (fat-equivalent, no marrow-replacing process)
- Symphysis and femoral heads

Lumbar spine
- Position:
  - Lumbar lordosis (sagittal survey image)
- Lumbosacral angle (see below)
- Bony spinal canal (shape, width—see below)
- Vertebral bodies (shape, margins, bone-marrow signal)
- Height of intervertebral disk spaces
- Intervertebral disks
- Dural tube

- Neuroforamina
- Nerve roots:
  - Origin and course
- Facet joints
- Vertebral arches intact
- Spinous processes
- Coccyx (shape, structure, position—see below)

Soft tissues
- Muscles (especially the iliac, psoas, gluteals, and intrinsic back muscles)
- Fat and intra-abdominal structures (e.g., sigmoid colon and rectum, bladder, prostate or uterus and ovaries)
- No masses

Vessels
- Aorta
- Iliac arteries
- Vena cava
- Iliac veins

Lymph nodes
- Lymph node stations (particularly the iliac nodes)

Important Data

1 Lumbosacral angle (S1/horizontal plane):
- 26–57°

2 Angle between sacrum and coccyx:
- Anterior angle ca. 10–30° (sagittal survey image, large range of variation)

3 Width of joint space:
- 4–5 mm

4 Articular cartilage:
- **a** Sacral: 3 mm
- **b** Iliac: 1 mm

Sagittal image

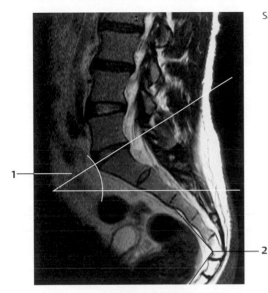

1 ——

—— 2

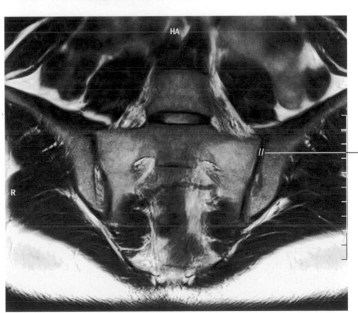

Paracoronal image parallel to the sacrum

—— 3

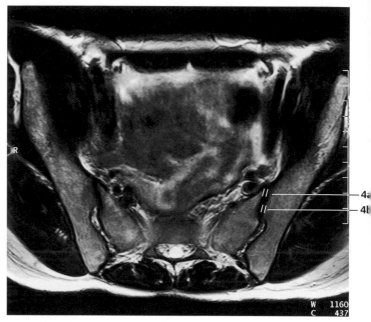

Para-axial image at right angles to sacrum

MRI: Joints

Temporomandibular Joint

The mandibular condyle has normal configuration and articulates with a normally shaped glenoid fossa.

The joint space is of normal width, and the articular surfaces have smooth, sharp borders. Cortical thickness and signal intensity of the bone marrow are normal.

The articular disk presents a hoodlike configuration on paracoronal images. It is dumbbell-shaped on parasagittal images. The posterior ligament is at approximatley the 11 o'clock position relative to the circumference of the mandibular condyle.

When the mouth is opened, the articular disk follows the movement of the mandibular condyle onto the articular tubercle.

Imaged portions of the paranasal sinuses are clear and pneumatized. Imaged portions of the neurocranium show no abnormalities.

Interpretation

The temporomandibular joint appears normal.

Checklist

Mandibular condyle
Glenoid

- Cylindrical shape (coronal plane)
- Spherical shape (sagittal plane)
- Shape (posteriorly convex, largely congruent with the mandibular condyle when the mouth is closed)
- Articular surfaces:
  - Margins (smooth, sharp)
- Joint space:
  - Width (see below)
  - No effusion
- Cortex:
  - Thickness
  - No subchondral changes
  - No osteophytes

	• Signal intensity of bone marrow (fat-equivalent)
	• No circumscribed signal changes
Articular disk	• Coronal plane:
	— Configuration (tubular or cylindrical)
	— Width (approximately uniform, 2–3 mm thick)
	— Position (surmounts mandibular condyle like a hood, does not project past medial or lateral aspect of condyle)
	• Sagittal plane:
	— Configuration (dumbbell-shaped: anterior ligament, intermediate zone, posterior ligament)
	— Position:
	— With mandible in resting position, posterior ligament is at about the 11–12 o'clock position relative to circumference of mandibular condyle
	— When mouth opens, articular disk moves with condyle (anterior ligament is anterior to condyle or at about the 11 o'clock position relative to condyle circumference) onto the articular tubercle
Surrounding soft tissues	• Muscles (particularly the masseter and lateral pterygoid)
	• Normal-appearing periarticular fat
	• No masses
	• No infiltration
Bony boundaries (skull base superiorly, external auditory canal and mastoid posteriorly)	• Smooth
	• Sharp
	• Intact
Adjacent structures (temporal lobe, mastoid process)	• Unremarkable
Paranasal sinuses (if imaged)	• Clear and pneumatized

Important Data

1 Posterior ligament:
- With jaw in resting position, between 11 and 12 o'clock

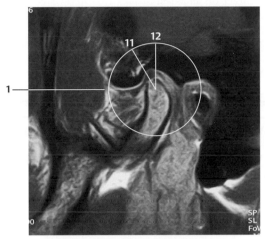

Parasagittal image with the mouth closed

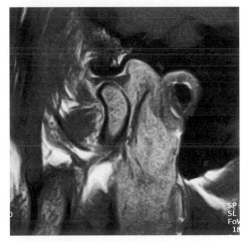

Parasagittal image with the mouth open

Shoulder Joint

The humeral head has normal configuration and articulates properly with the normally developed glenoid. The articular surfaces are smooth and show normal cortical thickness. The width of the joint space is normal. The bone marrow displays homogeneous, fat-equivalent signal intensity.

The glenoid labrum is intact on all sides.

The acromioclavicular joint has normal configuration, with no hypertrophy. The subacromial fat is intact.

The muscles comprising the rotator cuff show normal course and configuration. In particular, the supraspinatus muscle is normal in its position, width, and signal characteristics and shows a normal musculotendinous junction.

The intact biceps tendon appears normal and occupies a normal position in the bicipital groove.

The other muscles that cover the shoulder joint appear normal, as do imaged portions of the lungs and soft tissues.

Interpretation

The shoulder joint appears normal.

Checklist

Humeral head
- Position (centered in the shoulder joint; does not ride high in the glenoid)
- Configuration (rounded cross section). (Caution: the bicipital groove appears anteriorly and the tuberosity posteriorly, but the highest axial section is always circular—useful for excluding a proximal depressed fracture = Hill-Sachs lesion)
- Contours (smooth and sharp)
- No osteophytes, especially in fovea area
- Bone marrow signal:
  - Homogeneous, fat-equivalent intensity (in humeral head and shaft)
  - "Adolescent" bone marrow signal before age 25 years
  - No subchondral signal changes
  - Normal articular cartilage

Joint space
- Width (see below)
- No increase of intra-articular fluid

Glenoid	• Size congruent with humeral head
	• Smooth articular surface
	• Cortex (thickness, no discontinuities)
	• No osteophytes
	• No subchondral erosion
	• Bone marrow signal
	• Articular cartilage
	• Glenoid labrum is triangular about its whole circumference and is firmly attached to the glenoid. (Caution: variant often seen in the anterosuperior quadrant should not be mistaken for a tear!)
Acromion, clavicle	• Normal development of the acromion (straight, curved, hook-shaped, upslope angle—see below) and clavicle
	• Smooth, sharp margins
	• Normal bone-marrow signal
Acromioclavicular joint	• Configuration
	• Width (see below)
	• No hypertrophy
	• Normal subacromial fat layer
	• Subacromial bursa is not fluid-filled, fat stripe of bursa is visible and undisplaced
Rotator cuff (supraspinatus, infraspinatus, subscapularis, teres minor muscles)	• Configuration
	• Position
	• Course (over humeral head)
	• Homogeneous signal intensity of tendon
	• No hyperintense signal (on T2-weighted images)
	• No peritendinous fluid
Biceps tendon	• Long tendon segment runs in bicipital groove
	• Hypointense
	• No discontinuities
	• Normal width
	• No increase of fluid in long biceps tendon sheath
	• No fluid in other bursae (especially the subcoracoid and subdeltoid)
Muscles covering the shoulder joint (especially the deltoid)	• Shape
	• Position
	• Signal intensity
Lungs, soft tissues	

Important Data

1 Glenoid angle:
- Approx. 5° of retroversion (i.e., angle between the glenoid and a perpendicular to the scapular long axis is slightly open posteriorly, but the range of variation is large)

2 Joint space:
- Shoulder joint: < 6 mm

3 Acromioclavicular joint:
- Width < 1 cm

4 Angle of acromion upslope (oblique sagittal image plane):
- 10–40°

5 Diameter of biceps tendon:
- Approximately 4–6 mm

6 Bicipital groove:
- Width: 7–9 mm
- Depth: 4–7 mm

The bicipital groove starts at least 20 mm below the tip of the humeral head. (This differentiates the groove from a Hill-Sachs lesion, which often occurs at a higher level.)

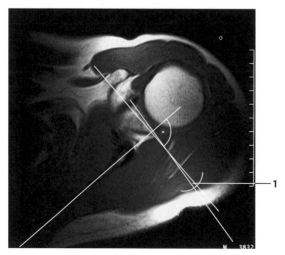

Axial image

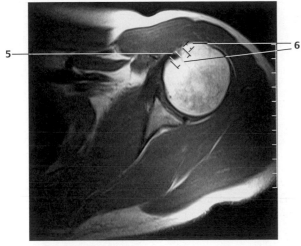

Axial image

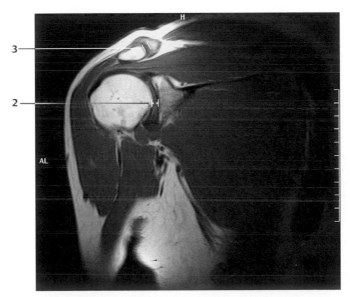

Paracoronal image parallel to the supraspinatus muscle

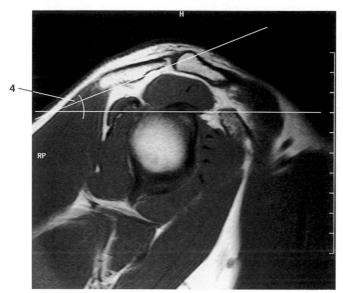

Parasagittal image at right angles to the supraspinatus muscle

Elbow Joint

The elbow joint shows normal configuration with normal articulation of the bone ends. The articular surfaces are smooth and congruent, especially in the radiohumeral and ulnohumeral joints, with no discontinuities. There are no osteophytes or subchondral joint changes.

The joint spaces are of normal width. The olecranon fossa is clear, and there are no intra-articular loose bodies.

The cortex of the tubular bones is of normal thickness. The bone-marrow signal is normal.

Imaged ligamentous structures appear normal, particularly the annular ligament.

The ulnar, radial, and median nerves display a normal course and diameter.

The imaged muscles show no abnormalities.

Interpretation

The elbow joint appears normal.

Checklist

Radius, ulna, humerus	• Normal configuration • Articulation • Position (see below)

Joint	• Articular surfaces are smooth and congruent, especially in the radiohumeral and ulnohumeral joints
	• Normal cortical thickness
	• No discontinuities in the articular surfaces
	• No marginal osteophytes
	• No subchondral joint changes
	• Normal olecranon fossa
	• Joint spaces:
	  — Width
	  — No loose bodies
	  — No effusion
	  — No synovial folds in radiohumeral joint

Cubital tunnel	• Shape • Depth • Retinaculum

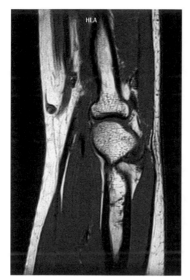

Sagittal image at level of radius

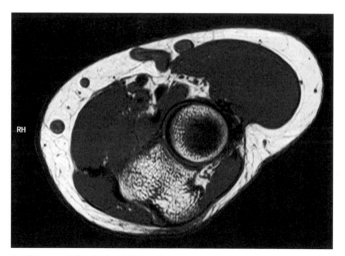

Axial image at level of radial head

Wrist

The bones comprising the wrist present a normal configuration.
The radial joint angle is normal. The carpal bones show normal shape
and relationship to one another and to the radiocarpal and carpometacarpal joints.

The articular surfaces are smooth and congruent with normal cortical
thickness and normal width of the joint spaces. There are no
osteophytes and no subchondral signal changes. The bone marrow signal is normal.

The ulnar (triangular) disk exhibits normal configuration and normal
signal characteristics. The interosseous ligaments also appear normal.

The carpal tunnel is of normal width and transmits tendons that are
normal in width and position. The median and ulnar nerves appear normal.

The metacarpals and phalanges have normal margins and normal bone-
marrow signal intensity. The soft tissues are normal.

Interpretation

The wrist and hand appear normal.

Checklist

Bony structures
- Radius
- Ulna (configuration, no shortening)
- Carpal bones (proximal and distal rows)
- Metacarpals
- Radiocarpal angle (see below)
- Carpal bones:
  - Shape and position (see below)
- Metacarpals and phalanges:
  - Five digital rays
  - Shape
  - Normal bone marrow signal
- Articular surfaces, especially of radiocarpal and
  carpometacarpal joints:
  - Smooth
  - Congruent
- Normal cortical thickness
- No marginal osteophytes
- No subchondral signal changes
- Normal width of joint space (see below)

Ligamentous structures	• Ulnar (triangular) disk:
	  — Configuration (see below)
	  — Margins
	  — Internal structure (hypointense expansion to styloid attachment and to radial end of ulna with central rarefaction)
	  — No signal abnormalities
	  — No discontinuities
	• Interosseous ligaments: scapholunate and lunatotriquetral ligaments and ligaments of the distal row of carpal bones
	  — Shape
	  — Signal intensity
	  — Contours (smooth, intact)
	• Extrinsic ligaments:
	  — Shape
	  — Signal intensity
	  — Contours (smooth, intact)

Carpal tunnel	• Width (see below) • Tendons (tendon sheaths in six compartments, thickness, position, symmetry) • Flexor retinaculum (no palmar convexity) • No circumscribed widening of tendons • No thickening of tendon sheath walls • No increase of fluid in tendon compartment • No fluid-filled cyst • No ganglion
Median nerve	• Course • Width • No impingement, especially in the carpal tunnel (axial image) • No diffuse or circumscribed swelling (e.g., common at level of pisiform bone) • No narrowing (e.g., common at level of hamate bone) • No signal changes
Ulnar nerve	• Width • Course • No expansion • No bony impingement
Soft tissues	• No subcutaneous nodules

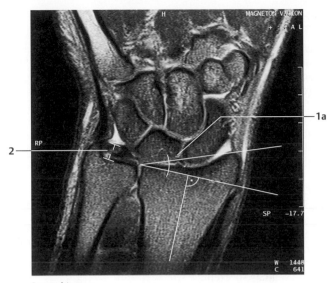

Coronal image

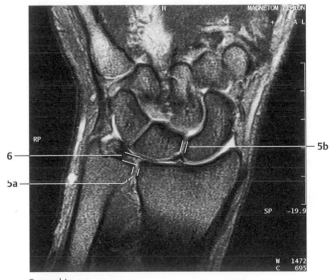

Coronal image

Important Data

1 **Radiocarpal angle:**
   a Coronal: 10–30°
   b Lateral: 10–15°
2 **Ulnar (triangular) disk or triangular fibrocartilage complex (TFC):**
   • Maximum thickness: 1.6 cm ± 0.5 cm
3 **Inclination of lunate bone relative to long axis (lateral view):**
   • 0–30°
4 **Inclination of scaphoid bone relative to long axis (sagittal view):**
   • 30–60°
5 **Joint spaces:**
   a Distal radioulnar joint: ca. 3 mm
   b Other joints: ca. 2 mm
6 **Distal radioulnar length relation:**
   • 1–5 mm
   • > 5 mm = ulnar shortening
   • < 1 mm = ulnar lengthening
7 **Lines are drawn tangent to the corners of the radial ulnar notch and to the base points of the roughly triangular cross section of the distal ulna. Lines are drawn perpendicular to these tangents, and the angle between them is measured:**
   • In neutral position +15° – +45°, in supination approx. +100°. Always compare with the opposite side.

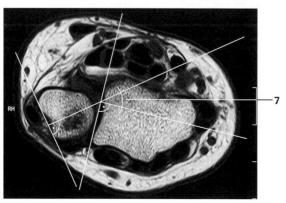

Axial image at level of distal radioulnar joint

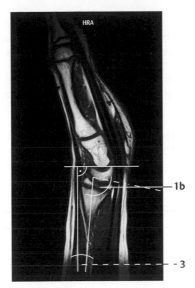

Sagittal image

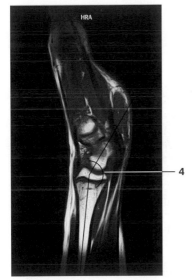

Sagittal image

Hip Joint

The femoral heads and acetabula are of normal shape, and the femoral heads are well covered by the acetabular margins. The joint spaces are of normal width.

The articular surfaces are smooth and congruent and show normal cortical thickness. There are no marginal osteophytes or subchondral signal changes.

The bone marrow shows normal signal intensity, especially in the femoral head and neck. Each femoral shaft has normal margins and contains a normal bone marrow signal.

The imaged muscles and the lesser pelvis show no abnormalities.

Interpretation

The hip joints appear normal.

Checklist

Hip joint
- Femoral heads:
  — Shape
  — Bilateral symmetry
- Acetabula:
  — Shape
  — Roundness
  — Symmetry
- Position:
  — Femoral heads articulate with the acetabula
  — Femoral heads are well covered by the acetabular margins (see below)
- Normal width of joint space
- Articular surfaces:
  — Contours (smooth and congruent)
- Normal cortical thickness on the articular surfaces
- No marginal osteophytes
- No subchondral signal changes
- Femoral head and neck:
  — Shape
  — Position
  — Normal femoral neck angle (CCD angle) (see below)

- Bone marrow signal:
  - Homogeneous
  - Fat-equivalent intensity
  - No circumscribed "double line sign" (femoral head necrosis) or patchy bone marrow edema

Other structures
- Femoral shaft:
  - Smooth margins
  - Normal cortical thickness
  - Bone marrow signal appropriate for age ("adolescent" signal before age 25) and homogeneous
- Musculature:
  - Anatomy
  - Course
  - Bilateral symmetry
  - Homogeneous signal intensity
  - No circumscribed hypointense or hyperintense areas
- Major nerves and blood vessels:
  - Course
  - No circumscribed expansion
- No lymphadenopathy
- Structures of the lesser pelvis (bladder, prostate, and seminal vesicles or uterus and adnexa, intestinal structures, lymph node stations)

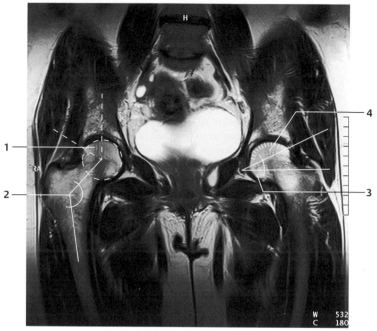

T2-weighted coronal image

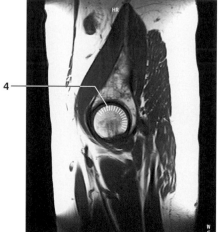

Sagittal image

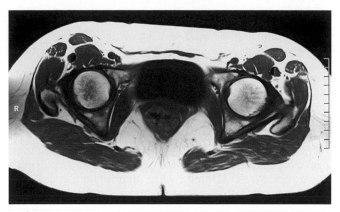

Axial image

Important Data

1 **Center-edge angle of Wiberg:**
   - 26–30°
2 **CCD angle:**
   - Approximately 125–135°
3 **Slope of acetabular roof:**
   - <10°
4 **Femoral head coverage by the acetabulum:**
   - Approximately 70% of articular surface

Knee Joint

The bones comprising the knee joint show normal configuration and position. The bone marrow signal is normal, with a normal trabecular pattern and normal epiphyseal lines.

The cortex shows smooth contours and normal thickness with no subchondral signal changes.

The cartilage covering the patella, femoral condyles, and tibial plateau is of normal thickness and has normal signal characteristics. The cartilaginous surface is smooth.

The medial and lateral menisci of the knee joint present a normal triangular configuration on axial images and have a homogeneous internal structure of low signal intensity. The anterior horn, midportion, and posterior horn each display a smooth, intact surface.

The anterior and posterior cruciate ligaments are intact and are normal in their width and signal characteristics. The collateral ligaments are intact and of normal width.

The soft tissues surrounding the knee joint and the imaged vascular structures are unremarkable.

Interpretation

The knee joint appears normal.

Checklist

Configuration and position	• Femur
	• Tibia
	• Fibula
	• Patella (shape, centering—see below)
Bone marrow signal	• Fat-equivalent
	• May be slightly patchy
	• Adolescent bone marrow signal before age 25 years
	• No bone marrow edema
	• No contusions
	• Normal trabecular pattern
	• Epiphyseal plate closure after age 18
Cortex	• Thickness
	• Contours (smooth)
	• No subchondral signal changes in the bone marrow

Articular cartilage (patella, femoral condyles, tibial plateau)	• Thickness (see below) • Signal characteristics • Cartilage surface (smooth)
Joint space	• Width • No effusion • No intra-articular foreign bodies • No abnormal synovial folds (especially the mediopatellar fold)
Medial and lateral menisci (anterior horn, midportion, posterior horn)	• Configuration (normal triangular cross section) • Internal structure (homogeneous, hypointense) • Contours (smooth, intact surface)
Anterior and posterior cruciate ligaments	• Continuity • Width • Course (see below) • Signal intensity (anterior cruciate ligament light and dark, posterior cruciate ligament uniformly dark)
Collateral ligaments	• Position • Width • Continuity • Low signal intensity
Soft tissues and imaged vessels	• No masses (e.g., Baker cyst, popliteal cyst, ganglion) • No varices

---

Important Data

Patella:
Shape: Wiberg I–III (see drawing)

Centering
1 **Patellar tilt angle** (formed by a line parallel to the lateral patellar articular surface and a line parallel to the posterior aspect of the femoral condyles [may be drawn in sections at various levels, if necessary]):
   • $> 8°$

2 **Congruence angle** (formed by the bisector of the notch angle and a line connecting the patellar apex with the deepest point of the notch):
  - 6° to -6°
3 **Notch angle:**
  - 135–145° (average ca. 138°)
4 **Lateral displacement:**
  - < 5% (i.e., less than 5% of the patella is lateral to a line that is perpendicular to the line joining the femoral condyles at the level of the lateral condyle)
5 **Patellar ligament:**
  a Length: 3.5–5.5 cm
  b Width: 2.5–3 cm
  c Thickness: 7 mm
6 **Ratio of length of patellar ligament to height of patella** = 0.8–1.2 (> 1.2 = high-riding patella)
7 **Cartilage:**
  a Patella: 3–4 ± 1 mm
  b Femoral condyles and tibial plateau: ca. 2.2 ± 0.6 mm

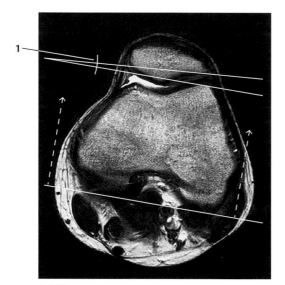

Axial image

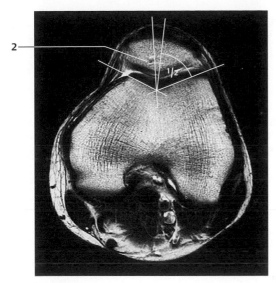

Axial image

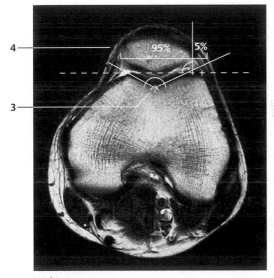

Axial image

8   Anterior cruciate ligament:
- Length: ca. 38 mm
- Width: ca. 11 mm
- **a** Angle formed by tangents to the tibial plateau and the anterior surface of the anterior cruciate ligament: 55°
- **b** Angle formed by Blumensaat's line (dashed) and the anterior surface of the anterior cruciate ligament: 1.6°
- **c** Angle of posterior cruciate ligament: ca. 123° (abnormal at ca. 106°)
- **d** Line of posterior cruciate ligament should intersect the distal femur.

Abnormal **c** and **d** are indirect signs of anterior cruciate ligament rupture.

Posterior cruciate ligament:
- Length: ca. 38 mm
- Width: ca. 18 mm

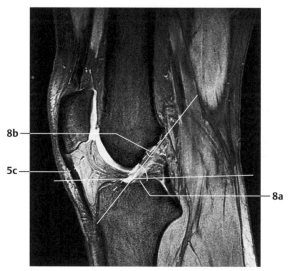

Sagittal image at the level of the anterior cruciate ligament

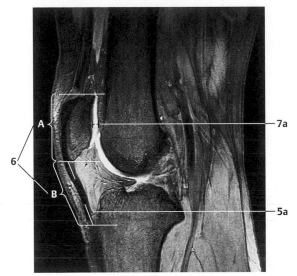

Sagittal image at the level of the patellar ligament

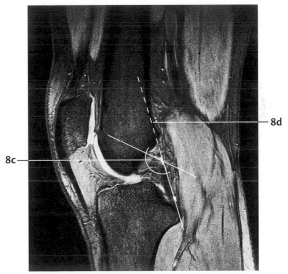

Sagittal image at the level of the posterior cruciate ligament

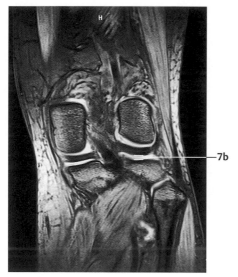

Coronal image

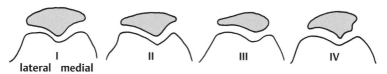

Wiberg classification of patellar shapes (right knee). (From Möller, T.B.: *Röntgennor-malbefunde*. Thieme, Stuttgart 1996.)

Ankle and Subtalar Joints

The bones comprising the ankle joint show normal position and configuration, with normal development of the ankle mortise.

The bone marrow signal, trabecular pattern, and epiphyseal lines are all normal.

The joint space is of normal width. The cortex shows normal thickness and smooth contours, especially along the tibial and talar articular surfaces. There are no subchondral signal changes and no osteophytes.

The lateral and medial ligaments are normal in their course, width, and signal characteristics.

The talocalcaneal and talonavicular joints appear normal. The interosseous ligament between the talus and calcaneus is intact. The Achilles tendon is normal in its course, width, and signal characteristics, and the preachilles fat is clear. The tendons and plantar aponeurosis are unremarkable.

The soft tissues show no abnormalities.

Interpretation

The ankle joint and subtalar joint appear normal.

Checklist

Skeleton	• Medial and lateral malleoli (ankle mortise), talus, calcaneus, tarsal bones:
	— Configuration
	— Position (shape, centering—see below)
	— Normal bone marrow signal
	— Epiphyseal plate closure after age 18
	— Normal trabecular pattern
Articular surfaces	• Congruence
	• Cortex:
	— Cortical thickness (uniform, no circumscribed expansion)
	• Contours: smooth and sharp, no subchondral signal changes (especially on the medial side = 60% site of predilection for osteochondritis dissecans), no discontinuities
	• Articular cartilage (if visible):
	— Thickness
	— Smooth surface

Ligaments	• Lateral ligaments (in order of trauma frequency: anterior fibulotalar ligament, fibulocalcaneal ligament, posterior fibulotalar ligament): — Course (not wavy) — Signal intensity — Width — Smooth contours — Continuity — No periligamentous fluid • Medial (deltoid) ligament: — Course — Signal intensity — Width (see below) — Smooth contours — Continuity • Interosseous ligament: — Course — Continuity • Achilles tendon: — Course — Width (see below) — Shape (transverse oval cross section) — Signal characteristics — Continuity (especially 2–6 cm above the calcaneal attachment = site of predilection for tears) — Normal-appearing preachilles fat
Subtalar joint (talocalcaneal joint, talonavicular joint)	• Configuration • Position • Width of joint space
Soft tissues	• Tendons: — Flexor hallucis longus tendon is particularly important (especially in the tarsal tunnel behind the medial malleolus, which is a site of predilection for tendinitis and rupture) — Tibialis posterior (its navicular attachment is a site of predilection for rupture) — Course — Signal intensity (uniformly hypointense, no central signal change) — Width — No discontinuities

- Wall of tendon sheath (no fluid increase or wall thickening)
- Plantar aponeurosis and calcaneonavicular ligament:
  - Shape
  - Width (see below)
  - Hypointense in all MRI sequences
  - No circumscribed expansion or nodularity
  - No subcutaneous edema
- Normal tarsal canal
- Soft tissues
- Blood vessels

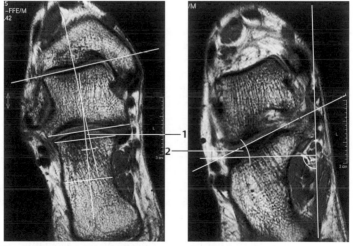

Fig. 1: Semicoronal image showing all of the posterior articular surface of the subtalar joint and portions of the medial and lateral malleoli

Fig. 2: Semicoronal image showing the posterior articular surface, all of the tarsal canal, and the sustentaculum

Important Data

Position

Semicoronal image plane:
1 **Calcaneal valgus angle** = relation of the talar axis (line connecting the bisectors of the corners of the ankle and subtalar joint surfaces) to the axis of the calcaneus (line connecting the bisectors of the corners of the subtalar joint and a line parallel to it through the narrowest part of the calcaneus):
   - Approximately 0° ± 10°
2 **Sustentacular angle** (formed by a line connecting the corners of the lateral posterior joint surface and sustentaculum and a line perpendicular to a tangent to the sustentaculum and medial calcaneal tuberosity):
   - 18–28°

Axial image plane (image is acquired 4 cm above the level where the lateral part of the talus is first visualized):
3 **Plantar talocalcaneal angle** (formed by a line connecting the lateral corner of the posterior articular surface of the talus and the medial corner of its medial articular surface with a line bisecting the calcaneal articular surface and the midpoint of a parallel line through the caudal third of the calcaneus):
   - 60–70°
4 **Calcaneocuboid angle** (angle between the longitudinal axes of the cuboid and calcaneus):
   - Approximately 20–35°
5 **Arch angle** (angle between tangents to the inferior calcaneal border and the soft-tissue sole):
   - 20–30°
6 **Achilles tendon:**
   - Anteroposterior diameter < 6 mm
7 **Lateral ligaments:**
   - Width of the anterior talofibular ligament and calcaneofibular ligament: 2–3 mm
   - Angle between the longitudinal axes of the first and second metatarsals = 7.4 ° ± 2.6° (> 9° is suspicious for hallux valgus)
   - Relation of calcaneus to talus: 1.8–2.1
8 **Boehler's angle** (formed by a line connecting the posterosuperior and anterosuperior prominences of the calcaneus and a line through the sustentaculum tali):
   - 20–40° (signifies calcaneal integrity)

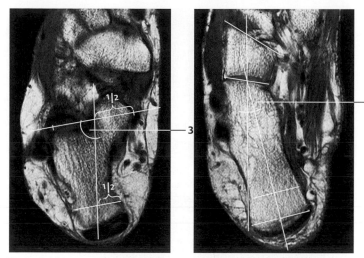

Fig. 3: Axial image 4 mm above the plane in which the lateral part of the tarsus is first visualized

Fig. 4: Axial image 8–10 mm above the plane in which the articular surface of the calcaneocuboid joint is first visualized

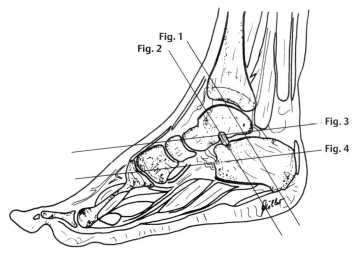

Location of the semicoronal and axial image planes

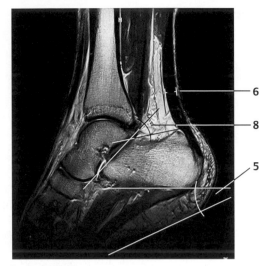

Sagittal image

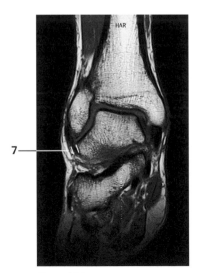

Coronal image

MRI: Special Investigations

Cranial Vessels

The internal carotid arteries show normal course and caliber and are symmetrically disposed. Each carotid siphon is normal, showing no displacement or extrinsic compression. Intraluminal signal intensity is homogeneous.

The middle cerebral artery arises normally from the internal carotid on each side and forms normal insular loops. There is no circumscribed vascular narrowing or dilatation. The vessel lumen shows homogeneous signal intensity.

The anterior cerebral artery shows no signs of narrowing or displacement.

The basilar artery shows a normal course and caliber and divides into normal-size posterior cerebral arteries. The anterior and posterior communicating arteries on each side are normally developed and of normal size. No segments show convolution or circumscribed dilatation.

The other evaluable portions of the neurocranium show no abnormalities.

Interpretation

The cranial vascular system appears normal.

Checklist

Internal carotid artery	• Extracranial portion • Siphon • Intracranial portion
Middle cerebral artery	• M1, M2, and M3 segments
Anterior cerebral artery	• Position (no displacement) • Course • Caliber (symmetry) • Signal characteristics (homogeneous intraluminal signal, no filling defect) • Contours (smooth, no circumscribed or beaded constrictions)

	• No circumscribed outpouching (especially in the proximal and horizontal segments)
Basilar artery	• Position
	• Course (no excessive tortuosity, no impression on brain stem)
	• Caliber (no general or circumscribed luminal dilatation)
	• Signal characteristics (homogeneous intraluminal signal, no filling defect)
	• Contours (smooth)
Posterior cerebral artery	• Position
	• Symmetry
	• Course
	• Caliber (symmetry)
	• Signal characteristics
	• No excessive tortuosity
	• No circumscribed dilatation, especially in the proximal segment
Anterior and posterior communicating arteries	• Presence
	• Course
	• Caliber
	• Signal characteristics
Venous vessels	• No arteriovenous communications
Neurocranium (imaged portions)	• No abnormalities

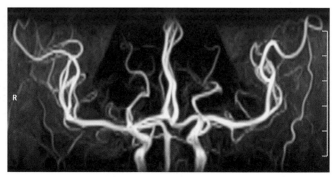

MR angiogram of the cranial arteries, coronal view

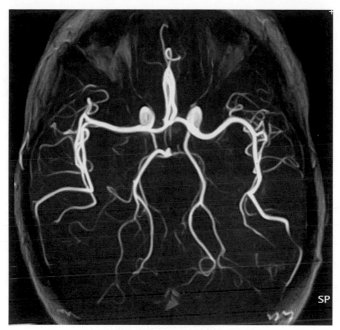

MR angiogram of the cranial arteries, axial view

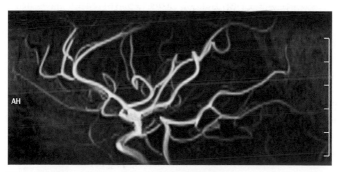

MR angiogram of the cranial arteries, lateral view

Cranial Venous Vessels

MRI of the venous cranial vessels demonstrates a superior sagittal sinus of normal caliber with normal arrangement of draining superficial cerebral veins. The great cerebral vein and inferior sagittal sinus appear normal. The transverse sinus presents a normal caliber and usually shows slight asymmetry between the right and left sides. The other evaluable deep cerebral veins are normally developed and patent. No venous segments contain flow voids or filling defects.

The other evaluable portions of the neurocranium show no abnormalities.

Interpretation

The cranial venous vascular system appears normal.

Checklist

Supratentorial venous system	• Superior sagittal sinus, superficial cerebral veins (ascending cerebral veins), deep cerebral veins:
	— Internal cerebral vein
	— Great cerebral vein (of Galen)
	— Straight sinus
	— Superficial middle cerebral vein
	— Sphenoparietal sinus
	— Cavernous sinus
	— Inferior petrosal sinus
	• Sinus confluence
	• Transverse sinuses (bilaterally symmetrical only in 20% of cases; 25% of cases have unilateral drainage, and more than 50% of cases show predominant right-sided drainage; bilateral asymmetry is normal, usually with a right-sided predominance)
	• Sigmoid sinus
	• Jugular bulb
Infratentorial venous system	• Position (no displacement)
	• Course (no excessive tortuosity, normal calibers, no general or circumscribed luminal dilatation)
	• Signal characteristics (homogeneous intraluminal signal, no filling defect)
	• Contours (smooth, no constrictions)

- No circumscribed outpouching
- No arteriovenous communications

Neurocranium • No abnormalities
(imaged portions)

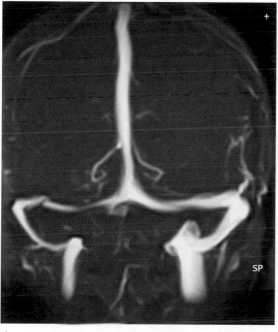

Phase-contrast angiogram of the cranial veins, anteroposterior view

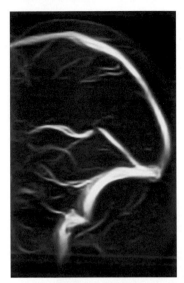

Phase contrast angiogram of the cranial veins, lateral view

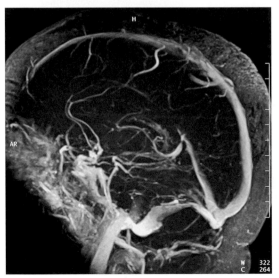

Contrast-enhanced maximum intensity projection (MIP) emphasizing the cranial veins, lateral view

MR Angiography of the Renal Arteries

The abdominal aorta displays normal course and caliber.
The renal arterial trunks are paired, arise at the proper level, and show normal distribution. The course, calibers, and contours of the renal vessels are normal, with no evidence of caliber irregularities.
The kidneys are paired and are normal in their position, shape, size, and borders.
Other imaged vessels show no abnormalities.

Interpretation

The renal arteries appear normal.

Checklist

Abdominal aorta	• Position (almost straight course slightly to left of midline)
	• Bifurcation (see below)
	• Diameter (see below)
	• No caliber irregularities
	• No circumscribed or segmental narrowing
Renal arteries	• Number (paired)
	• Accessory polar arteries
	• Origin from the aorta (see below)
	• Further distribution (anterior and posterior main branches, segmental arteries)
	• Diameter (see below)
	• No caliber irregularities (circumscribed, segmental, beaded)
	• No pathological vessels
	• No stretching or splaying
Renal paren-chyma	• Paired renal organs
	• Position (see below)
	• Size (see below)
	• Smooth organ contours
Renal pelvis	• Structure
	• Bilateral symmetry
	• Width
	• Shape of calices
Ureters	• Not duplicated (one per side)
	• Course

- Diameter (see below)
- No obstruction of urinary drainage

Other imaged vessels (e.g., iliac vessels, spinal arteries, superior and inferior mesenteric arteries)
- Course
- Caliber (see below)

Venous phase (if documented, e.g., inferior vena cava and renal veins)
- Course
- Caliber (see below)

Important Data

1 **Abdominal aorta:**
- Approximately 18–30 mm

2 **Aortic bifurcation:**
- At approximately the L4-L5 level

3 **Origin of renal arteries:**
- At approximately the L1-L2 level

4 **Renal artery:**
- Diameter approximately 4–10 mm

5 **Position of superior poles of kidneys:**
   a Right: superior border of L1
   b Left: inferior border of T12 (right kidney is lower than left kidney by up to one vertebral body height)

6 **Distance between superior renal poles:**
- Approximately 10 cm (4–16 cm)

7 **Distance between inferior renal poles:**
- Approximately 13 cm (9–18.5 cm)

8 **Renal dimensions:**
- Craniocaudal: 8–13 cm (<1.5 cm craniocaudal difference in renal sizes)

   Renal cortical thickness:
- 4–5 mm

   Time to corticomedullary equilibrium:
- 1 minute

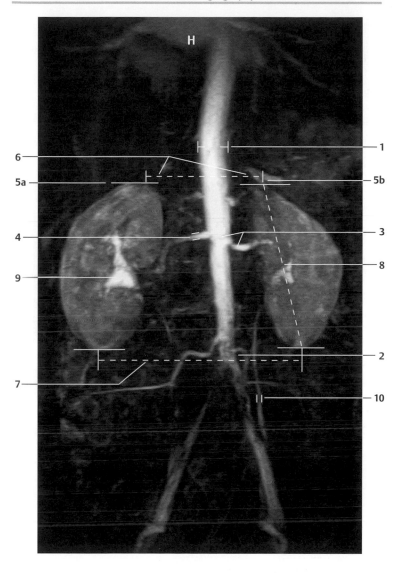

9 Contrast excretion into the pyelocaliceal system:
- 3 minutes

10 Width of ureter:
- 4–7 mm

Inferior vena cava:
- Transverse diameter up to 2.5 cm

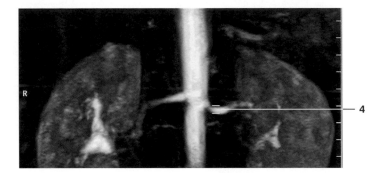

Pelvic and Lower Limb Vessels

The abdominal aorta is normal in its course, diameter, and filling.
The aortic bifurcation occurs at a normal level, with normal visualization of the common, internal, and external iliac arteries.
Both common femoral arteries have normal calibers, smooth walls, and a homogeneous intraluminal signal. The femoral arteries show a normal course, caliber, and distribution.
The superficial femoral artery appears normal, especially within the adductor canal. Like the popliteal artery, the vessel shows a normal course and no irregularities in its caliber. It divides normally into the three lower leg arteries, which show normal course, caliber, and distribution.

Interpretation

The vascular system of the pelvic and lower limb arteries appears normal.

Checklist

Vascular course and caliber (described from center to periphery)

- Abdominal aorta:
  - Position: slightly to left of midline
  - Almost straight course
  - Bifurcation (see below)
- Common iliac artery
- External iliac artery
- Internal iliac artery
- Common femoral artery
- Superficial femoral artery (see below)
- Circumflex femoral artery
- Profunda femoris artery
- Popliteal artery (see below)
- Anterior tibial artery
- Posterior tibial artery
- Peroneal (fibular) artery:
  - Position (no displacement)
  - Course (no excessive tortuosity or coiling)
  - Caliber
  - Signal characteristics (homogeneous intraluminal signal, no filling defect)

- Contours (smooth; no circumscribed, segmental or beaded constrictions; particularly note superficial femoral artery in the adductor canal)
- No circumscribed outpouching (e.g., popliteal artery)

Veins
- No arteriovenous communications

Vessels
- No pathologic vessels or cutoffs

Soft tissues and bony structures
- (If evaluable)

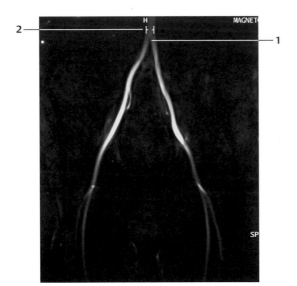

Phase-contrast angiogram of the pelvic vessels

Important Data

1 Bifurcation:
- At approximately the L4-L5 level

Vascular calibers:

2 Abdominal aorta:
- Approximately 2–4 cm

3 Superficial femoral artery:
- Approximately 0.7–1.5 cm

4 Popliteal artery:
- Approximately 0.6–1 cm

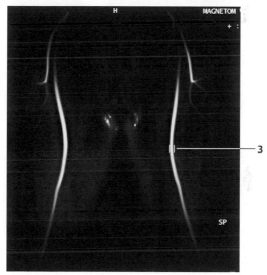

Phase-contrast angiogram of the femoral vessels

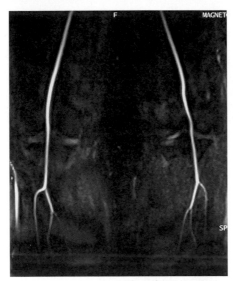
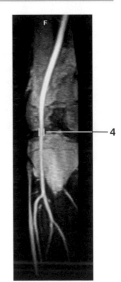

Phase-contrast angiogram of the vessels about the knee joints

MR Cholangiopancreatography

The common bile duct shows normal position, caliber, and length with a homogeneous, fluid-equivalent intraluminal signal. The cystic duct and imaged portions of the intrahepatic bile ducts also appear normal. The gallbladder is of normal size; it has smooth borders and homogeneous contents.

The pancreatic duct shows normal position, length, and caliber with homogeneous internal structure and smooth contours.

Interpretation

The bile ducts, gallbladder, and pancreatic duct appear normal.

Checklist

Common bile duct	• Course:
	   — Usually slightly convex toward the left side
	• Size:
	   — Tapers slightly from its origin (the right and left hepatic ducts and common hepatic duct are of equal size)
	   — No circumscribed caliber irregularities, especially in the papillary area (e.g., prestenotic dilatation, discrete or segmental stenosis due to tumor or fibrosis)
	   — No circumscribed narrowing (stricture) or dilatation
	• Shape:
	   — Contours (smooth, straight)
	   — Number (one)
	• Internal structure:
	   — Homogeneous fluid-equivalent signal intensity
	   — No calculi
	   — No tumor

Gallbladder	• Position • Number (one) • Shape • Possible septation • Size (see below)

- Contours:
  - Smooth
  - Straight
  - No diverticula
- Internal structure:
  - Homogeneous fluid-equivalent signal
  - No filling defect (sludge, stone, papilloma, carcinoma)

Cystic duct and intrahepatic bile ducts
- Position (presence and number)
- Course
- Size
- Contours
- Filling

Pancreatic duct
- Position:
  - Horizontal
  - Ascends toward left side
- Size:
  - Diameter tapers uniformly toward the duodenum
  - No circumscribed change in diameter (e.g., constriction by a tumor, cyst, or inflammation; prestenotic dilatation due to a tumor; segmental ectasia such as the segmental irregularities in pancreatitis)
- Shape:
  - Contours (smooth with straight walls)
  - No irregular margins
  - Not sacciform
  - Not tortuous or dilated
- Internal structure:
  - Homogeneous fluid-equivalent signal
  - No calculi
  - No tumor

Important Data

1 Gallbladder:
- Horizontal diameter up to 5 cm (> 5 cm is suspicious for hydrops)

2 Width of common bile duct:
- ≤ 8 mm (after cholecystectomy: ≤ 10 mm)

3 Cystic duct:
- Length ca. 4 cm

4 Pancreatic duct:
- Width: 1–3 mm

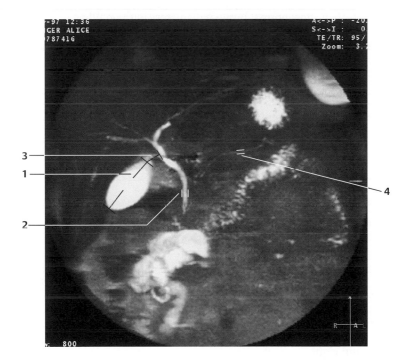

Cervical Arteries

The aortic arch presents smooth walls and normal configuration.
The brachiocephalic trunk arises normally and undergoes a normal division into the subclavian artery, common carotid artery, and right vertebral artery. The left common carotid artery arises directly from the aortic arch, has a normal caliber, and shows no luminal narrowing or filling defects. The vertebral artery appears normal.
The carotid bifurcation occurs at a normal level on each side and is normally shaped. The external carotid artery and particularly the internal carotid artery are symmetrical on each side and have normal calibers. There is no circumscribed narrowing or expansion.
The vessels display a homogeneous intraluminal signal. The carotid siphon appears normal, showing no displacement or extrinsic compression.
The vertebral arteries are symmetrically disposed and take a normal course. They show normal luminal diameters with no filling defects or caliber irregularities as far as the basilar artery.
The portions of the neck that are imaged and evaluable show no abnormalities.

Interpretation

The supra-aortic system of arterial cervical vessels appears normal.

Checklist

Aortic arch	• General form
	• Course
	• Caliber
	• Signal characteristics
	Origins: brachiocephalic trunk, left common carotid artery, left subclavian artery
Brachiocephalic trunk	• Origin
	• Division into right subclavian and right common carotid arteries
Left and right subclavian arteries	• Position
	• Course
	• Caliber
	• Signal characteristics

Common carotid artery	• Origin (usually the left artery arises directly from the aortic arch while the right artery arises with the subclavian artery from the brachiocephalic trunk)
	• Symmetry
	• Course
	• Caliber (symmetry)
	• Signal characteristics
	• No excessive tortuosity
	• No circumscribed dilatation
Carotid bifurcation	• Usually occurs at C4/5 or C3/4 level
	• Shape
	• No circumscribed narrowing, especially at the origin of the internal carotid artery
Internal carotid artery	• Position (no displacement)
	• Course
	• Caliber (slight proximal dilatation due to the carotid sinus, right–left symmetry)
	• Signal characteristics (homogeneous intraluminal signal, no filling defect)
	• Contours (smooth, no circumscribed constriction or ulceration)
	• No circumscribed narrowing (especially in the proximal segment) with poststenotic dilatation
	• Symmetrical appearance of the carotid siphons
External carotid artery	• Position
	• Course
	• Caliber
	• Signal characteristics
Vertebral artery	• Origin (from the subclavian artery or, rarely, from the aortic arch)
	• Position
	• Course (no excessive tortuosity)
	• Caliber (no general or circumscribed luminal dilatation)
	• Caliber discrepancy (usually left > right) is common
	• Signal characteristics (homogeneous intraluminal signal, no filling defect)
	• Contours (smooth)

Important Data

Sites of predilection for stenosis:
- Internal carotid artery:
  — Carotid bifurcation (ca. 2/3 of all carotid stenoses)
  — At entrance to the carotid siphon
  — Within the carotid siphon
- Vertebral artery
  — Origin from the subclavian artery
  — Passage through dura at craniocervical junction

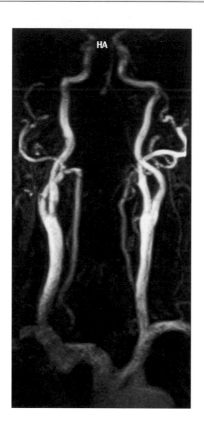

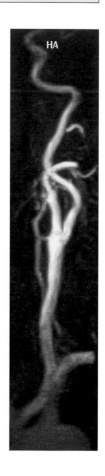

References

Allen, K. S., H. Y. Kressel, P. P. Arger, H. M. Pollack: Age-related changes of the prostate: evaluation by MR Imaging. Amer. J. Roentgenol. 152 (1989) 77–81

Berli, A., R. Putz, M. Schumacher: Maße und Varianten im Bereich des Canalis opticus. Radiologe 32 (1992) 436–440

Biggemann, W., W. Frobin, P. Brinckmann: Physiologisches Muster lumbaler Bandscheibenhöhen. Fortschr. Röntgenstr. 167 (1997) 1

Brown, H. K. et al.: Uterine junctional zone: correlation between histologic findings and MR Imaging. Radiology 179 (1991) 409–413

Buthiau, D., D. L. Kaech: CT und MR in der klinischen Praxis. Huber, Bern 1996

Chan, T. W., M. K. Dalinka, J. B. Kneeland, A. Chervrot: Biceps tendon dislocation: evaluation with MR Imaging. Radiology 179 (1991) 649–652

Claussen, C., B. Lochner: Dynamische Computertomographie. Springer, Berlin 1983

Dähnert, W.: Radiology Review Manual. Williams & Wilkins, Baltimore 1996

Dihlmann, W.: Computertomographie des lumbalen Diskusprolapses und der Vertebralkanalstenose. Z. Rheumatol. 43 (1984) 153–159

Elster, A. D.: Modern imaging of the pituitary. Radiology 187 (1993) 1–14

Frahm, R., E. Drescher: Topographische Anatomie, Radiologie und Pathologie der Handwurzel und des Handgelenkes. Schnetztor, Konstanz 1988

Frahm, R., H. Fritz, E. Drescher: Winkelmessung des Rückfußes im CT. Fortschr. Röntgenstr. 151 (1989) 77–81

Friedmann, G., E. Büchelei, P. Thurn: Ganzkörper-Computertomographie. Thieme, Stuttgart 1981

Gentili, A., L. L. Seeger, L. Yao, H. M. Do: Anterior cruciate ligament tear: indirect signs at MR Imaging. Radiology 193 (1994) 835–840

Graßhoff, H., C. Buhtz, I. Gellerich, Ch. v. Knorre: CT-Diagnostik bei der Instabilität des Schultergelenkes. Fortschr. Röntgenstr. 155 (1991) 523–526

Gürtler, K.-F., R. W. Janzen, J. Hageman, H. F. Otto: CT des Mediastinums bei Myastenia gravis pseudoparalytica. Fortschr. Röntgenstr. 136 (1982) 35–40

Hamm, B., T. Römer, M. Albig, R. Felix, K.-J. Wolf: Magnetische Resonanztomographie der Ovarialtumoren. Fortschr. Röntgenstr. 146 (1987) 429–438

Harnsberger, H. R.: Handbook of Head and Neck Imaging. Mosby, St. Louis 1995

Hosten, N., Ch. Schubert, M. Cordes, R. Schneider, R. Felix: Kernspintomographie der Orbita bei endokriner Orbitopathie. Röntgenpraxis 41 (1988) 400–405

Hübener, K.-H.: Computertomographie des Körperstammes. Thieme, Stuttgart 1985

Jend, H.-J., H.-Ch. Tödt: Arbeitsbuch Computertomographie. Schnetztor, Konstanz 1989

Kahn, Th.: Leber-Galle-Pankreas. Thieme, Stuttgart 1996

Klaue, K., C. W. Durnin, R. Ganz: The acetabular rim syndrome. J. Bone Jt Surg. B 73-B (1991) 423–429

Kock, C.: Sagittale Weiten des cervikalen Wirbelkanales im Computertomogramm. Radiologe 26 (1986) 239–241

Lange, S.: Niere und ableitende Harnwege. Thieme, Stuttgart 1993

Lee, M. J., W. Mayo-Smith, P. Hahn, M. Goldberg, G. Boland, S. Saini, N. Papanicolaou: MR Imaging of the adrenal gland. Radiographics 14 (1994)

Lörcher, U., H. Schmidt, K. H. Hering: HR-CT der Lunge. Thieme, Stuttgart 1996

Maier, W.: Hochauflösende CT des Pankreas. In Bargon, G.: Symposium über bildgebende Verfahren in der Pankreasdiagnostik. Schnetztor, Konstanz 1986

Maier, W.: Zur Wertigkeit der Nativ-CT bei der akuten Pankreatitis. Fortschr. Röntgenstr. 150 (1989) 458–461

Möller, T. B.: Röntgennormalbefunde, 2, Aufl. Thieme, Stuttgart 1996

Möller, T. B., E. Reif: MR-Atlas des muskuloskelettalen Systems. Blackwell, Berlin 1993

Möller, T. B., E. Reif: Taschenatlas der Einstelltechnik, 2. Aufl., Thieme, Stuttgart 1995

Möller, T. B., E. Reif: Taschenatlas der Schnittbildanatomie, Bd. I, 2. Aufl., Thieme, Stuttgart 1997

Moore, S. G., G. S. Bisset III, M. J. Siegel, J. S. Donaldson: Pediatric musculoskeletal MR Imaging. Radiology 179 (1991) 345–360

Mühlberger, V.: Kardio-CT. Röntgenpraxis 39 (1985) 329–352

Munk, P. L., C. A. Helms: MRI of the Knee. Lippincott-Raven, Philadelphia 1996

Murphey, M. D., L. H. Wetzel, J. M. Bramble, E. Levine, K. M. Simpson, H. B. Lindsley: Sacro iliitis: MR Imaging findings. Radiology 180 (1991) 239–244

Nugent, R. A. et al.: Graves orbitopathy: correlation of CT and clinical findings. Radiology 177 (1990) 675–682

Outwater, E. K., D. G. Mitchell: Normal ovaries and functional cysts: MR appearance. Radiology 198 (1996) 397–402

Pickuth, D.: Sonographie – systematisch. Bon-Med, Lorch 1993

Pommeranz, S.: Gamuts & Perls in MRI. MRI-EFI Publications, Cincinnati 1993

Putz, R.: Anatomie des Retroperitonealraumes: In Frommhold, P., P. Gerhard: Tumoren im Retroperitonealraum. Klinisch-radiologisches Seminar, Bd. 16. Thieme, Stuttgart 1987

Reiser, M., M. Nägele: Aktuelle Gelenkdiagnostik. Thieme, Stuttgart 1992

Richards, R. D., D. J. Sartoris, M. N. Pathria, D. Resnick: Hill-Sachs lesion and normal humeral groove: MR Imaging features allowing their differentation. Radiology 190 (1994) 665–668

Robertson, P. L., M. E. Schweitzer, A. R. Bartolozzi, A. Ugoni: Anterior cruciate ligament tear: evaluation of multiple signs with MR Imaging. Radiology 193 (1994) 829–834

Schild, H. H., F. Schweden: Computertomographie in der Urologie. Thieme, Stuttgart 1989

Schneider, B., J. Laubenberger, M. Wildner, V. Exne, M. Langer: Kernspintomographisches Messungsverfahren von Femurantetorsion und Tibiatorsion. Fortschr. Röntgenstr. 163 (1995) 229–231

Schumacher, K. A., J. M. Friedrich: Die Computertomographie in der Diagnostik der Nierenerkrankungen. In Bargon, G.: Symposium über bildgebende Verfahren in der Diagnostik der Nieren und oberen Harnwege. Schnetztor, Konstanz 1987

Scotti, G. et al.: MR Imaging of cavernous sinus involvement by pituitary adenomas, Amer. J. Roentgenol. 151 (1988) 799–806

Scoutt, L. M. et al.: Junctional zone of the uterus: correlation of MR Imaging and histologic examination of hysterectomy specimens. Radiology 179 (1991) 403–407

Smith, D. K.: Anatomic features of the carpal scaphoid: validation of biometric measurements and symmetry with tree-dimensional MR Imaging. Radiology 187 (1993) 187–191

Stern, E. J., C. M. Graham, W. R. Webb, G. Gamsu: Normal trachea during forced expiration: dynamic CT measurements. Radiology 187 (1993) 27–31

Stiskal, M., A. Neuhold, R. Weinstabl, F. M. Kainberger, B. Gisinger: MR-tomographische Befunde bei Achillodynie. Fortschr. Röntgenstr. 153 (1990) 9–13

Sugimoto, H., T. Shinozaki, T. Ohsawa: Triangular fibrocartilage in asymtomatic subjects: investigation of abnormal MR signal intensity. Radiology 191 (1994) 194–197

Sugimura, K., B. M. Carrington, J. M. Quivey, H. Hricak: Postirradiation changes in the pelvis: assessment with MR Imaging. Radiology 175 (1990) 805–813

Takashi Ohnishi, et al.: Levator palpebrae superioris muscle: MR evaluation of enlargement as a cause of upper eyelid retraction in graves diseases. Radiology 188 (1993) 115–118

Tomczak, R. et al.: Messung des femoralen Torsionswinkels von Kindern durch MR im Vergleich zu CT und Ultraschall. Fortschr. Röntgenstr. 163 (1995) 224–228

Uhlenbrock, D.: MRT und MRA des Kopfes. Thieme, Stuttgart 1996

Vahlensieck, M., M. Reiser: MRT des Bewegungsapparats. Thieme, Stuttgart 1997

Vannier, M. W. et al.: Brain surface cortical sulcal lengths: quantification with three-dimensional MR Imaging. Radiology 180 (1991) 479–484

Wegener, O. H.: Ganzkörpercomputerto-mographie. Blackwell, Berlin 1992

Wiesen, E. J., J. R. Crass, E. M. Bellon, G. G. Ashmead, A. M. Cohen: Improvement in CT Pelvimetry. Radiology 178 (1991) 259–262

Woerner, H., G. Brill, T. Frenzel, H. Stoll, M. Tesseraux: Pelvimetrie mittels Kern-spintomographie. Fortschr. Röntgenstr. 149 (1988) 378–382

Zaunbauer, W., S. Däpp, M. Haertel: Anat-omische Normalmaße im zervikalen Computertomogramm. Radiologe 25 (1985) 521–524

Index